Parish Nurses,
Health Care Chaplains,
and Community Clergy
Navigating the Maze
of Professional Relationships

THE HAWORTH PRESS
New, Recent, and Forthcoming
Titles of Related Interest

Broken Bodies, Healing Hearts: Reflections of a Hospital Chaplain by Gretchen W. Tenbrook

A Practical Guide to Hospital Ministry: Healing Ways by Junietta Baker McCall

Parish Nursing: A Handbook for the New Millennium by Sybil D. Smith

When Life Meets Death: Stories of Death and Dying, Truth and Courage by Thomas William Shane

Shared Grace: Therapists and Clergy Working Together by Marion Bilich, Susan Bonfiglio, and Steven Carlson

Faith, Spirituality, and Medicine: Toward the Making of the Healing Practitioner by Dana E. King

The Pastor's Guide to Psychological Disorders and Treatments by W. Brad Johnson and William L. Johnson

In the Shadow of Our Steeples: Pastoral Presence for Families Coping with Mental Illness by Stewart D. Govig

Parish Nurses, Health Care Chaplains, and Community Clergy

Navigating the Maze of Professional Relationships

Larry VandeCreek, DMin
Sue Mooney, BSN
Editors

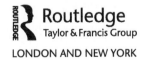

Routledge
Taylor & Francis Group

LONDON AND NEW YORK

First published by
The Haworth Press, Inc.
10 Alice Street
Binghamton, N Y 13904-1580

This edition published 2011 by Routledge

Routledge
Taylor & Francis Group
711 Third Avenue
New York, NY 10017

Routledge
Taylor & Francis Group
2 Park Square
Milton Park, Abingdon
Oxon OX14 4RN

PUBLISHER'S NOTE
Identities and circumstances of individuals discussed in this book have been changed to protect confidentiality.

Cover design by Anastasia Litwak.

Library of Congress Cataloging-in-Publication Data

Parish nurses, health care chaplains, and community clergy : navigating the maze of professional relationships / Larry VandeCreek, Sue Mooney, editors.
    p. cm.
Includes bibliographical references and index.
    ISBN 0-7890-1617-6 (alk. paper)—ISBN 0-7890-1618-4 (soft)
    1. Parish nursing—United States. 2. Nurses—Professional relationships. 3. Chaplains, Hospital—United States. 4. Chaplains, Hospital —Professional relationships. 5. Clergy—United States. 6. Clergy—Professional relationships. I. VandeCreek, Larry. II. Mooney, Sue F. Dromgoole.

RT120 . P37 P365 2002
259' .4—dc21

2002069070

CONTENTS

SECTION III: PREPARATION FOR PARISH NURSING—SPIRITUAL FORMATION AND CLINICAL PASTORAL EDUCATION

SECTION IV: INTERPROFESSIONAL DYNAMICS

Chapter 9. How to Begin a Parish Health Ministry: A Juggling Act

Joyce Kaatz
Tammy Anderson
Valerie Putnam
Don Lehmann

Chapter 10. Invitation to a Shared Community Ministry

Judy Raley
Barbara Weinhold

Chapter 11. Spiritual Care: Bridging the Disciplines in Congregational Health Ministries

Karen Hahn
James M. Radde
John E. Fellers

SECTION VII: FURTHER COOPERATION AND RESOURCES FOR GROWTH

ABOUT THE EDITORS

Larry VandeCreek, DMin, retired as Director of Pastoral Research at the HealthCare Chaplaincy, Inc. in New York City on June 30, 2001. Dr. VandeCreek is a member of numerous professional associations including the Association of Professional Chaplains, Inc., the American Association of Pastoral Counselors, and the Association for Clinical Pastoral Education. He has published many journal articles and abstracts, and is the author of "A Research Primer for Pastoral Care and Counseling" (*Journal of Pastoral Care Publications,* 1988) and editor of *Scientific and Pastoral Perspectives on Intercessory Prayer* (Haworth, 1998). In addition, he is the co-editor of *The Chaplain-Physician Relationship* (Haworth, 1991), *Ministry of Hospital Chaplains: Patient Satisfaction* (Haworth, 1997), and *The Discipline for Pastoral Care Giving: Foundations for Outcome Oriented Chaplaincy* (Haworth, 2001). Dr. VandeCreek received his Doctor of Ministry degree from Trinity Lutheran Seminary in Columbus, Ohio, his Master of Theology in Pastoral Counseling from the Columbia Theological Seminary in Atlanta, Georgia, and his Master of Divinity from Calvin Theological Seminary in Grand Rapids, Michigan.

Sue Mooney, BSN, earned her degree from The Ohio State University and a compelled unit of clinical pastoral education at Grant/Riverside Methodist Hospital in Columbus, Ohio. She is a parish nurse in the Overbrook Presbyterian Church in Columbus. Mooney is a Health Minister Consultant for the Presbyterian Church (USA), a member of the denomination's Parish Nurse Task Force, and part of the leadership team for the Presbyterian Health Network. She has led over 100 workshops locally and nationally on parish nursing.

CONTRIBUTORS

Tammy Anderson, RN, is Parish Nurse, First Presbyterian Church and Avera McKenna Hospital, Sioux Falls, South Dakota.

Larry Austin, DMin, is Director of Pastoral Services, Pitt County Memorial Hospital, Greenville, North Carolina.

Lindsay B. Carey, M App Sc, is National Research Officer for the Australian Health and Welfare Chaplains Association and Associate Lecturer, School of Public Health, La Trobe University, Melbourne, Victoria, Australia.

Margaret B. Clark, DMin, is Teaching Chaplain, Pastoral Care Services, University of Alberta Hospital, Edmonton, Alberta, Canada.

Paul Derrickson, MDiv, is Coordinator of the Department of Pastoral Services, the Milton S. Medical Center, Hershey, Pennsylvania.

Pamela K. Evans, RN, is Parish Nurse, First Presbyterian Church, Derby, Kansas, and a member of the nursing faculty, Butler County Community College, El Dorado, Kansas.

John E. Fellers, DD, is Executive Director, the Institute of Religion, Houston, Texas.

Pat Fosarelli, MDD, DMin, is Professor of Spirituality, Parish Nursing, and Pastoral Theology at the Ecumenical Institute of Theology and Assistant Professor of Pediatrics, Johns Hopkins School of Medicine, Baltimore, Maryland.

Dan Magnus Geeding, DMin, is a staff chaplain in the Department of Pastoral Care, Waukesha Memorial Hospital, Waukesha, Wisconsin.

Richard B. Gilbert, BCC, is Executive Director of the World Pastoral Care Center and Connections and Director of Pastoral Care at Shuman Hospital, Elgin, Illinois.

Karen Hahn, MSN, is Executive Director of the Center for Faith and Health Initiatives, Houston, Texas.

Dorothea Honn, BSN, MDiv, is a parish nurse, First United Methodist Church, Waukesha, Wisconsin.

James C. Johnson, MDiv, is Health Care Chaplain, Mercy General Health Partners, Muskegon, Michigan.

Joyce Kaatz, MS, RN, is Parish Nurse, Home Health Services, Our Savior's Lutheran Church and Sioux Valley Hospital and University Medical Center, Sioux Falls, South Dakota.

William R. Leety, BD, is Pastor of Overbrook Presbyterian Church, Columbus, Ohio.

Don Lehmann, MDiv, is Pastor of Caring Ministries, Our Saviour Lutheran Church, Sioux Falls, South Dakota.

Joan L. Murray, MN, DMin, was Associate Professor, Chaplaincy Services and Pastoral Education, University of Virginia Health System, Charlottesville, Virginia. She is now Director of Chaplaincy Services, Memorial Sloan-Kettering Cancer Center, New York, New York.

Joanne K. Olson, RN, PhD, is in the College of Nursing, University of Alberta, Edmonton, Alberta, Canada.

Linda L. Pape, MSN, is Parish Nurse Program Coordinator, Grant/ Riverside Methodist Hospitals, Columbus, Ohio.

Valerie Putnam, RN, DMin, is Senior Pastor, Westminster Presbyterian Church, Sioux Falls, South Dakota.

James M. Radde, SJ, MDiv, is Health Care Chaplain Educator, Minneapolis, Minnesota.

Judy Raley, MA, is with Memorial Health Care System, Chattanooga, Tennessee.

Dawn B. Rigney, RN, PhD, is Assistant Professor, University of Virginia School of Nursing, Charlottesville, Virginia.

Renae Schumann, RN, PhD, is Assistant Professor, University of Texas Houston Health Science Center, Houston, Texas.

Judith Allen Shelly, RN, DMin, is Editor of the *Journal of Christian Nursing,* Frederick, Pennsylvania.

Sybil D. Smith, PhD, is a consumer advocate, Family and Community Health, Lyman, South Carolina.

Sandra Thomas, DMin, is Director, Partners in Parish Nursing, Millersville, Maryland.

Tim VanDuivendyk, DMin, is Director of Chaplaincy Services, Memorial Hermann Healthcare System, Houston, Texas.

Anne Van Loon, RN, PhD, is Founding Chairperson and Director of Development of the Australian Faith Community Nurses Association and Lecturer in Nursing, Flinders University, Adelaide, South Australia.

Barbara Weinhold, MSN, is with Memorial Health Care System, Chattanooga, Tennessee.

Preface

Almost everyone knows that health care systems are changing. Health care financial reform efforts sharply curtail physician and hospital expenditures and this influences the provision of care in at least two ways. First, getting the attention of physicians is increasingly difficult unless one is seriously ill. For example, the routine annual physical examination has markedly changed during the last fifteen years. Examinations are now more cursory, more rapid; previously established routine procedures disappear as physicians try to cope with restricted payments from managed care companies. The logic is simple: lower payments for medical services contribute to less medical attention.

The second change concerns hospitalization. Many medical procedures previously requiring hospitalization are now conducted on an outpatient basis and patients are more seriously ill before being admitted to the hospital. It is increasingly more difficult to be admitted to the hospital. Beyond that, it is more difficult to remain in the hospital; patients are discharged more quickly.

Although these changes in the medical system seek to generate financial savings, they also create other consequences. Patients and their family members are more frequently "on their own," left to cope as best they can. Three examples illustrate these consequences. How are previously healthy patients to cope when they are sent home the day after surgery? They may have few persons locally who can come to their aid. Spouses may care for young children and hold full-time jobs. Or again, how are the chronically ill, particularly those with limited medical knowledge and financial resources, to contend with diminished medical attention? How are patients with chronic, extensive heart disease or cancer to behave when their busy physician tells them at the end of their visit to "just call if you have a problem," rather than instructing them to arrange for their regular return appointment? Finally, the old and frail have increasing problems with curtailed medical attention. They may suffer from dementia, have no means of transportation to medical appointments, and lack the attention of family members who live far away. How are they to cope with their increasing infirmities? Such situations are associated with greater morbidity, mortality, and the increased frustration of all involved.

Parish nurses (or "congregational nurses" or "faith community nurses") step into the vacuum. They are often registered nurses (RNs) with a significant personal religious history who join a church staff, either as volunteers or in paid positions, full- or part-time, and provide services that focus on the intersection of health, faith, and spirituality. Thus, parish nurses represent the concerns of the congregation for its members who are coping with health problems. In many ways, the parish nurse movement is a response to health care reform; congregations are saying, "We will take care of our own," although sometimes this ministry also extends to others outside the congregation.

The parish nurse movement is not without its problems, however. Parish nurses must navigate a maze of professional and organizational relationships that may not be wholly open to receiving them. While the need for parish nurses is evident, what are parish clergy (or "community clergy," "congregational clergy," or "faith community clergy") to think when a nurse seeks to join the church staff? Some clergy do not link religious faith and practice to health concerns; they turn interested nurses away. Some clergy are professionally threatened because they sense that nurses could become competitors. Others wonder how they can oversee such a health-related ministry.

Still, it is even more professionally and organizationally complex. Health care chaplains (or "hospital chaplains"), the professional siblings to both community clergy and parish nurses, often think of hospital patients as their parishioners. They frequently have ambivalent relationships with community clergy who make pastoral visits in the hospital, and the ambivalence can escalate when parish nurses begin to make such visits as well. It seems logical that health care chaplains, parish nurses, and community clergy would cooperate in providing care for those in need, but this cooperation can be difficult to achieve.

Two dynamics further confound this relationship triangle. First, as hospitals fight for their market share of patients, administrators quickly realize that parish nurses can be their ideal allies in the community. They understand that parish nurses are legitimized by religious congregations, can direct patients to their hospitals, and provide follow-up care after discharge. This seems a winning combination for all involved—except that clergy and congregations (or "parishes" or "faith communities") may wonder if they are being used by hospitals for commercial advantage. How can congregations and commercial health care institutions relate to each other? All persons involved in these professions need to think clearly about these interrelationships.

The second dynamic that complicates relationships concerns the clinical supervision of parish nurses. Parish nurses are, professionally speaking, out in the community by themselves without on-site medical or nursing supervision. Some parish nurses lack training in outpatient care, having left acute health care settings in frustration over health care reform. Who will help them learn the skills of a ministry involving outpatient nursing? In addition, always in the background is the specter of professional liability insurance coverage. Certainly community clergy and hospital chaplains cannot supervise the nursing aspects of their ministry. Some hospitals offer a solution: they provide arrangements for clinical supervision of the parish nurse through designated personnel who promote parish nursing in the community. Once again, however, such a quid pro quo arrangement merits examination. What are the assumptions involved in such arrangements?

In summary, the interprofessional relationships of parish nurses, health care chaplains, and community clergy present complex challenges that must be navigated if congregants and others in the community are to receive the care they need. Parish nursing is a new profession that is likely to grow because its roles and functions make intuitive sense in the confusing world of health care. But how are relationships to be built and managed? These are the concerns addressed in this book.

We assume that not all readers are familiar with the ministries of parish nursing and health care chaplaincy. The book begins with chapters that introduce each profession in Section I. Evans, herself a parish nurse, describes parish nursing, focusing on seven aspects of the profession. Johnson, a board-certified chaplain, writes about health care chaplaincy, emphasizing professional training in the first principles of spiritual reality, faith development, and emotional process.

The ministry of parish nursing must certainly rest on theological foundations. In Section II, Allen Shelly presents a Christian theology of nursing, tracing the development of the nursing profession out of the early and medieval Christian church. Her description of modernist, postmodernist, and biblical theologies merits attention from all interested parties. Credentialed as a nurse and serving as a chaplain, she reports that some patients are more spiritually open to her when she works as a nurse than when she functions as a chaplain.

Five chapters in Section III describe preparation for parish nursing. Thomas writes about a spiritual formation program as part of parish nursing course work. Some parish nurses report that clinical pastoral education is helpful and three chapters, including one from a Canadian setting, discuss its processes and curriculum. Two programs were explicitly designed for parish nurses. Murray and Rigney identify how they built a parish nursing training institute at a major university.

Section IV contains four chapters that describe interprofessional dynamics. Two parish nurses and two community clergy portray starting a parish nurse program as similar to a juggling act. Raley and Weinhold invite the three professions to engage in a shared ministry that can provide a holistic approach to the spiritual needs of congregations. Hahn, Radde, and Fellers identify the professional, legal, relational, and theological role definitions of the three professions, giving examples of role violations as well. Van Loon and Carey report the development of faith community nursing in Australia, drawing interesting parallels and contrasts to the situation in the United States.

Section V contains descriptions of three practice models in four chapters. The section begins with a description of working relationships within a church staff involving a parish nurse in a Midwest Presbyterian church. In the first chapter, the clergy and parish nurse discuss how they conceptualize their ministry and how they work together. This is followed by an edited telephone interview that involves the two of them as well as two associate pastors, thereby providing a broader perspective on how the church staff manages relationships. The third chapter, by authors in Texas, relates their collaborative efforts; their goal is to "help people be better, feel better, and carry suffering better." The section closes with a chaplain and a parish nurse reporting how they built an interprofession group within the hospital that increased attention to the spiritual needs of patients and family members.

Section VI focuses on the relationships of the three professions to health care agencies. Pape, who coordinates a parish nursing program for a large Midwestern hospital, discusses her role and function, particularly how the resources of the hospital provide supervision for parish nurses in the community, which is appealing to both clergy and congregations. Smith steps back from these practical details and provides a "theoretical lens" through which to view the foundations of parish nursing programs and their relationships to health care agencies. She promotes a clearer understanding of the foundations upon which the three professions can build firm relationships.

Both chapters in the last section reach outward. Fosarelli, a physician and theology teacher, hopes that physicians can also join this team effort. She pleads for less professional territorialism in the interest of helping patients. Gilbert provides an annotated bibliography with emphasis on aging, bereavement, care of the sick, counseling for emotional support, and domestic violence.

Changes in health care systems provoke many additional changes, some of which we noted at the beginning of this preface. Professional relationships also change. We offer this book to all who are thinking about parish nursing, about the relationship of these three professions, and about how the people of God can receive the health and spiritual care they need.

SECTION I:
INTRODUCTION TO PARISH NURSING
AND HEALTH CARE CHAPLAINCY

Chapter 1

Who Are Parish Nurses?

Pamela K. Evans

Who are parish nurses? This simple question requires a somewhat complex answer. In many ways, the profession is still in its formative stages. Its professionals possess a variety of educational preparations and come from diverse health care backgrounds. They bring with them the uniqueness of their individual faith and strong interpersonal skills. Their practice is shaped by the Nurse Practice Act of each state and guided by the scope and standards of practice. Several practice models are beginning to emerge. This discussion briefly describes these considerations.

VARIED PROFESSIONAL BACKGROUNDS

The education and previous clinical experience of parish nurses influence how they perceive their role and the skills they bring to their practice. Some come from hospital-based specialty areas, including medical-surgical, obstetrical, pediatric, psychiatric, critical care, and emergency nursing. Nurses from general medical-surgical areas will bring knowledge of adult health care related to illness and surgery. These RNs may have specialized experience in such areas as cardiology, head and spine, or cancer. Those coming from an obstetrical background have a wealth of knowledge in the care of mothers and babies during pregnancy, delivery, and postdelivery. Pediatric nurses work with the care of children from infancy until the age of eighteen or twenty-one years. In large health care centers, pediatrics may be further divided into all of the specialty areas found in adult care. Psychiatric nursing involves the care of individuals, either adults or children, with mental disturbances. Critical care nursing involves the care of individuals in all of the specialty intensive care units, including an understanding of highly technical equipment. Emergency nursing is the care given in the trauma unit, including accident victims and the ill child or adult seeking care and hospital admission. Many of these nursing specialties require rapid decision making under close supervision.

Those nurses coming from nonhospital settings may include office nursing, home health, community health, and nursing education. Office settings range from primary care settings to minor surgery centers. Home health nursing involves all of the care and treatment provided in the home. Community health nursing involves the planning and care of groups of persons within the community.

Other nonhospital nurses include those working in the varied levels of long-term care and nursing education. In the past, long-term care (LTC) typically involved the elderly but now includes younger persons who need more care than can be provided in the home setting. Parish nurses who come from nursing education likely have previous experience in a variety of health care settings. They have completed advanced education in nursing and chosen to spend their time and energies in the education of future nurses. Indeed, parish nurses come to this ministry from these wide-ranging areas of the profession.

Variety of Education

Parish nurses come from a variety of educational backgrounds. Basic nursing education for years involved the diploma, hospital-based, three-year curriculum. Although a few states continue to offer such diploma programs, the majority of nurses who graduate today hold an associate degree (AND) or bachelor's degree (BSN) in nursing. The AND degree is usually completed in a two-year community college setting, generally having thirty to forty credit hours of nursing and the remainder in sciences and general education. The BSN degree consists of a basic educational program in a four-year college or university and includes forty to fifty credit hours in nursing, the sciences, and the liberal arts.

Advanced degrees in nursing include the master's level (MS, MSN, MN) and the doctoral level (DNS, PhD). These nurses have chosen a variety of special emphasis areas in their graduate degrees. If they have chosen advanced licensure, they may hold an advanced registered nurse practitioner (ARNP) degree. Depending on state laws, they may then practice at different levels of independence.

Licensed practical nurses (LPNs) or licensed vocational nurses (LVNs) who completed a one-year vocational technical school may work with the RN in parish nursing. The practice roles of the LPN and RN are defined by the Nurse Practice Act of the individual state. Generally the LPN works under the direction of the RN.

The field of parish nursing as a new area is evolving from a variety of preparations. A few master's programs offer a parish nurse track. Some nurses choose clinical pastoral education (CPE) as a means of preparing themselves; various CPE programs for parish nurses are described later in this volume. Other nurses obtain their preparation in seminars and workshops; twenty states require continuing education for licensure renewal (American Nurses Association [ANA], 1999). Still others pursue self-study courses or distance education programs. Then others just do it without special training. The ANA first recognized parish nursing as a specialty in 1998 (HMA/ANA).

Each Parish Nurse Is Unique

Parish nurses bring a rich and varied background to their new ministry context. Many graduated from diploma programs administered by church-owned facilities; the curricula in these programs frequently gave attention to spiritual concerns. Many have twenty to thirty years of clinical practice and a maturity grounded in their faith communities. These nurses tend to understand spiritual development processes.

Nurses must have strong interpersonal skills that facilitate their relationships with patients and family members. For example, the obstetrical nurse is present at the joyous birth of a child but also must support the family when that infant dies or is born with a birth defect. The pediatric nurse must support the family after the physician has related the severity of the child's illness. Nurses in other areas often support the patient or family when the illness or death of a loved one is shared.

These interpersonal skills are also required in today's complex health care team. Many specialized physicians and therapists may see hospital patients. The nurse often serves as interpreter and coordinator between the treatment team members, patients, and their family members.

The parish nurse draws on these interpersonal skills to assist congregational members in negotiating the complex health care resources available in the community. These interpersonal skills are also called on in relating to the local church staff and judicatory staff members of denominations.

A PERSONAL STORY

The author has chosen to share her personal/professional journey in nursing as an example of personal uniqueness that is valued in parish nursing. I graduated from a diploma (Methodist) school of nursing in the mid-1960s. As was common then, I married immediately following graduation and worked in the obstetric department at the medical center that housed my school until the birth of our first child. While my husband was overseas I worked in a family practice office and then returned to being a "full-time mom." As our two children reached school age I returned to work part-time in maternal/child areas of the same facility. During this time we continued an active role in our local church (Presbyterian), both serving as church officers. In the late 1970s, as the diploma nursing programs closed, I returned to the local university to complete my BSN. Following its completion, I entered nursing education (ADN) and completed my MN.

During the early 1980s I read an article on parish nursing in our denomination's publication and was intrigued but did not pursue it. A few years later I asked of our local pastor if he was aware of parish nursing but again I did not follow up. In 1992 our adult daughter was diagnosed with cancer, and while with her, I read that her church (Methodist) was beginning a parish nurse program. The knowledge of the support of these parish nurses eased the difficulty of my returning home and leaving her 800 miles away. Following her death in 1993, I received a brochure on a seminar exploring development of parish nursing in the state, sponsored by the Methodist Conference in 1994. It was exciting to attend this seminar and find over 200 nurses and pastors present to explore parish nursing.

This seminar gave me the opportunity to explore the parish nurse preparation that was available at that time: (1) a series of seminars for nurse-pastor teams hosted by the Methodist Conference, (2) a master's in health ministry available from a school of theology 200 miles away, and (3) a distance learning program (DLP) based in Wisconsin. Our pastor was undergoing treatment for cancer at that time so the team program was not realistic for us. I explored his support of my joining the DLP; he enthusiastically gave it, partly because he had previously served as a hospital chaplain. The DLP I chose (Missouri Synod Lutheran) involved extensive directed readings and activities, as well as close work with a parish nurse mentor and with my pastor. Following an agreement of support from our local church board, I enrolled in the DLP. The community college where I am employed granted me a sabbatical for the fall of 1994, which allowed me to work on my parish nurse program. I was able to complete the DLP by January 1995 when I returned to my position on the nursing faculty. I have continued my parish nurse practice on a part-time nonsalaried basis since that time. In June 1995 and 2000, I attended national seminars on parish nursing sponsored by the Presbyterian Church (PCUSA), given my denominational ties. In 1997 the local Roman Catholic medical center started a parish nurse network that met monthly for information and support; it hosted conferences in 1998 and 1999 for spiritual and professional growth. In 1999, we began a network of Presbyterian parish nurses in our local area.

RESOURCES

Suggested resources for those who wish to explore parish nursing include books, journals, workshops or seminars, and the Internet (Table 1.1). Books of interest include Westberg (1990) and Solari-Twadell, Djupe, and McDermott (1990) and the Health Ministries Association (HMA)/ANA (1998) practice standards for parish nurses. Journals to explore include *Journal of Christian Nursing* and denominational journals. Check with local health care and educational facilities for workshops and seminars. A recent search of the Internet identified over 100 sites for "parish nursing," some of which describe local congregations, educational facilities, interfaith health programs, and the International Parish Nurse Resource Center. Check with denominational resources for established parish nurse programs and support.

TABLE 1.1. Resources for Parish Nursing

Books		
Title	**Author**	**Source**
Scope and Standards of Parish Nursing Practice	HMA/ANA	American Nurses Publishing <www.nursingworld.org>
Parish Nursing: The Developing Practice	Solari-Twadell	Parish Nurse Resource Center
Parish Nursing: Promoting Whole Person Health Within Faith Communities	Solari-Twadell	Sage Publications
The Parish Nurse	Westberg	Parish Nurse Resource Center

Journals
Journal of Christian Nursing, Box 1650, Downers Grove, IL 60515

Sample Internet Sites	
Page	**URL**
Center for Congregational Health Ministry	http://www.via-christi.org/cchmweb.nsf/mainview
Interfaith Health Programs	http://www.ihpnet.org
Augustana College	http://www.augie.edu/dept/nurs/marya.htm
Parish Nurse Concentrate	http://www.capital.edu/nursing/nursmsnparish.htm
Parish Nursing	http://www.synodofcovenant.org.HMPN.html
International Parish Nurse Resource Center	http://www.advocatehealth.com/about/faith/pn.ursctr.htm
Congregational Health Ministry	http://www.lcms.org/bhcm/hm/pn.htm
Division for Church in Society	http://www.elca.org/dcs/healthmin.html

Limitations

Nurses, health care chaplains, and community clergy who wish to explore development of parish nurse programs are encouraged to undertake a series of steps. First, check for practice limitations stipulated by the local state's Nurse Practice Act, which can be purchased from the State Board of Nursing (SBN). In most instances, the National Council of State Boards of Nursing Internet Web site (www.ncsbn.org) will provide linkage to the state board. The Nurse Practice Act delineates the role and practice of nurses by licensure, i.e., RN, ARNP, and LPN. Each nurse is held responsible for knowing the practice act of the state(s) in which he or she is licensed and practicing. *Caution: Do not use an unlicensed nurse.* The purpose of licensure is to protect the public.

Second, secure a copy of *Scope and Standards of Parish Nursing Practice* (HMA/ANA, 1998). This can be purchased from the ANA through their Web site (www.nursingworld.org/index.htm) or possibly from the local state or district nurses association.

Third, review the church's liability insurance for coverage of staff and volunteers in this role. Individual nurses should also check with their insurance providers for coverage. Parish nurse preparation programs will generally issue a certificate of completion that can be helpful when obtaining coverage. ANA has recognized parish nursing as a specialty and it is expected that certification will follow. Some denominations are developing their own certification for health ministry.

Parish nurses whose faith persuasion differs from the congregation in which they serve encounter occasional problems. These may include sacramental issues related to infant baptism versus believer's baptism, and whether these nurses can assist in serving communion to shut-ins (Mueller, 1999). Other issues might arise concerning end-of-life decisions and the termination of pregnancy. In general, parish nurses will have already dealt with their responses to such problems earlier in their nursing career. The clergy and parish nurse need to address such issues before service begins.

Another concern arises when non–faith-based institutions launch parish nurse programs. Their emphasis is often on the role of the nurse rather than the person served. These programs tend not to emphasize the integration of faith and health; they are market-driven and are often connected to managed care. Ministry/mission models are driven by a love of God and service to the congregation, in which the nurse is seen as a lay minister (Smith, 1999).

HISTORY OF PARISH NURSING

Parish nursing recognizes Dr. Granger Westberg as its founder. As a new clergy in a university town, he had the opportunity to experience hospital chaplaincy and observe closely the nursing role in caring for the whole individual—body, mind, and spirit. While teaching religion and health he developed a case study presentation format of physician, nurse, and pastor, symbolizing a rare form of patient care. From this experience he realized that nurses could bridge the gap between the sciences and humanities. With the help of a W. K. Kellogg Foundation grant, he, with others, set up medical offices in church buildings with teams comprised of doctor, nurse, and clergy. From this grew the concept of the parish nurse in the congregation (Westberg, 1990).

In 1984-1985, Westberg started a program of salaried nurses within the churches through Lutheran General Hospital in Chicago. This began as a partnership between six churches and the hospital. During the first two years of the project, the five roles of parish nurse were defined as (1) health educator, (2) health counselor, (3) coordinator of volunteers, (4) liaison with the community, and (5) integrator of faith and health (Solari-Twadell, Djupe, and McDermott, 1990).

This work then spread from the Chicago area to rural areas of Iowa where access to health care requires extensive travel. In 1988, the Evangelical Lutheran Church in America (www.elca.org/dsc/health min.html) became a partner and by 1998 had programs in 804 congregations. Since that time, parish nursing has spread throughout the United States and Canada, as churches and denominations react to health care as big business. They have reclaimed their role in the health and wholeness of their members. In 1999, Koch reported an "estimated 2,500 nurses working in some form of health or parish ministry." One example of its growth is the Center of Congregational Health Ministry (1999) established in 1997 that now lists parish nurses in 158 congregations representing twenty-two denominations in thirty-seven communities in south central Kansas and north central Oklahoma (http://www.via-christi.org/cchmweb.nsf/mainview?openview).

TYPES OF PRACTICE

The types of parish practices are closely related to the skills and abilities of individual nurses as well as the needs and resources of the congregation. For example, the practice of a parish nurse in a large inner-city congregation will likely differ from one in a rural setting. The nurse will likely emphasize referral and advocacy if extensive health care resources are available nearby. If health care resources are more limited, education and support may be the major roles. The nurse in a large congregation may need specific office hours; those in smaller congregations may rely on the telephone. One clinical service that seems common in most parish nurse programs is blood pressure screening for the congregation.

At least two models of parish nursing are available: congregation-based and institution-based. Congregation-based parish nurses serve as members of the ministry staff of an individual congregation and report to the pastor and boards of the local church. Here the nurses provide services to members of the congregation. In institution-based models, a nurse relates to the congregation through the local hospital that provides education and support.

Parish nurses may be salaried or unsalaried. Salaried parish nurses may be employees of a health care facility or nursing school whose time is purchased by the local congregation or they may be employed by the congregation. At issue here is that experienced nurses' salaries may approach that of the pastor of smaller congregations, and not be within the church's financial means. In some instances several congregations share a salaried parish nurse coordinator. Unsalaried parish nurses may also be based solely in the local congregation or associated with a local health care institution that provides education and support.

In summary, this material has introduced the basic structures of parish nursing to those who wish to explore it further. Many of the issues briefly presented here must be seriously considered before beginning a program.

REFERENCES

American Nurses Association (ANA). (1999). States that Require HIV/AIDS Continuing Education. <http://www.nursingworld.org/gova/hivceu.htm>.

Center of Congregational Health Ministry (1999). Churches with Parish Nurses. <http://www.via-christi.org/cchmeweb.nsf>, accessed September 27, 2000.

Health Ministries Association (HMA)/ American Nurses Association (ANA). (1998). *Scope and Standards of Parish Nursing Practice.* Washington, DC: American Nurses Publishing.

Koch, M.W. (1999). Nursing Leadership in Faith Community. *Worldwide Nurse.* <http://wwnurse.com/Nurse-zine>.

Mueller, H. (1999). Counselor's Corner. *Parish Nurse, A Newsletter by and for Parish Nurses in Service to a Christian Health Ministry.* 8(4), p. 3.

Smith, S.D. (1999). Parish Nursing, a Call to Integrity. *Journal of Christian Nursing, 17*(1), pp. 18-20.

Solari-Twadell, P.A., Djupe, A.M., and McDermott, M.A. (1990). *Parish Nursing: The Developing Practice.* Park Ridge, IL: Lutheran General Health Care System.

Westberg, G. (1990). *The Parish Nurse.* Minneapolis, MN: Augsburg Fortress.

Chapter 2

An Introduction
to Health Care Chaplaincy

James C. Johnson

This chapter provides an introduction to the unique role of health care chaplains. Their professional expertise and special responsibility involve bringing the resources of religion and faith to the support of a person's spirit with the aim of promoting health in the whole of the individual's life—body, mind, spirit, and relationships. One of the early leaders (Dicks, 1996/1940) in the development of the profession put it well:

> The chaplain is interested in the patient's recovery of physical health, and . . . will do anything he can to aid that recovery. . . . He is further interested in the spiritual growth of the patient: he knows that in suffering and stress people are either thrown back or else they gain confidence in the fundamental nature of things and it is the chaplain's hope to steady and aid them in any way that he can during such stress. (pp. 4-5)

According to Gillman and colleagues (1996), this means that

> the role of the chaplain is to relate to the other, whether patient, family, or other partner-in-care, as a whole person with a particular focus on spiritual or religious needs. . . . religious needs may include the request for prayer, sacraments or ritual, talking about one's relationship with God, or establishing contact with one's faith community. . . . spiritual needs include searching for meaning in the face of crisis, identifying and accessing one's inner resources for strength, reformulating one's spiritual identity

in the face of disruption, developing effective coping strategies, and finding healing in the midst of brokenness. (p. 11)

Handzo (1996) adds, "Regardless of the patient's ethnic, religious, or cultural background, the chaplain can address these issues, both in terms of the common human experience and with an informed perspective on and reverence for the specifics of the patient's background" (p. 45).

The Joint Commission on Accreditation of Healthcare Organizations (JCAHO) recognizes the importance of this aspect of health care: "for many patients, pastoral counseling and other spiritual services are an integral part of health care and daily life" (1997, RI 14). It mandates that

> hospitals respect and provide for each patient's right to pastoral counseling [and notes that] clinical chaplains assess and treat patients using individual and group interventions to restore or rehabilitate spiritual well-being. Clinical chaplains counsel individuals who are experiencing spiritual distress, as well as their families, caregivers, and other service providers, about their spiritual dysfunction or the management of spiritual care. (1997, RI 15)

The focus on spiritual health by chaplains can be further clarified by looking at two concepts: spiritual well-being, which the chaplain seeks to promote, and the nursing diagnosis of spiritual distress, which the chaplain seeks to alleviate.

SPIRITUAL WELL-BEING/SPIRITUAL DISTRESS

Spiritual well-being is defined as the "affirmation of life in a relationship with a higher power (as defined by the person), self, community, and environment that nurtures and celebrates wholeness" (Carpenito, Mondoux, and Waterhouse, 1995, p. 903). Indicators of spiritual well-being include the following:

- An awareness of the sacred
- Self-consciousness
- A unified inner core

- Inner peace and inner strength
- Commitment to and motivation by ultimate values
- A sense of meaning and purpose in life
- Acceptance of the past and hope for the future
- Trust and harmony in relationships
- The ability to love
- Appreciation of beauty and truth
- A relationship with the transcendent or a higher power or God
- A sense of humor (Adapted from Carpenito, Mondoux, and Waterhouse, 1995; Kim, McFarland, and McLane, 1995)

Current research indicates that spiritual well-being is an essential and integral component of general well-being (Levin and Larson, 1997; Larson, Swyers, and McCullough, 1998). Thus, chaplains supporting the faith of individuals and enhancing their spiritual health has a positive impact on their general health status.

In health care facilities where they work, chaplains accomplish this by addressing spiritual distress.[1] Spiritual distress is defined as "a disruption of the life principle which pervades a person's entire being and which integrates and transcends biopsychosocial nature" (Gordon, 1982, p. 226). This condition may often occur in the health care setting and is readily diagnosed by health care professionals. Since pastoral care "staffing levels usually do not permit 'making rounds' on all new patients to assess spiritual needs . . . , most chaplains rely on staff members for referrals and for guiding them to persons who have an acknowledged or suspected need" (Wagner and Higdon, 1996, p. 18). Therefore, it is very important that physicians, hospital nurses, allied health care providers, parish nurses, and local clergy recognize spiritual distress. Its indicators include these:

- Anger toward God (as defined by the person)
- Displacement of anger (especially toward religious representatives)
- Questioning the meaning of suffering
- Questioning the meaning of one's own life
- Questioning the ethical implications of treatment
- Verbalization or other display of inner conflicts
- Ambivalence about beliefs

- Request for spiritual assistance
- Demonstration of discouragement or despair
- Expression of a sense of emptiness
- Display of emotional detachment
- Nightmares or sleep disturbance
- Alteration of behavior or mood evidenced by crying, withdrawal, preoccupation, anxiety, hostility, apathy, fearfulness, etc.
- Self-blame
- Denial of responsibility
- Somatic complaints
- Gallows humor (Adapted from Carpenito, Mondoux, and Waterhouse, 1995; Kim, McFarland, and McLane, 1995)

Such "disturbance in the belief or value system that provides strength, hope, and meaning to life" (Carpenito, Mondoux, and Waterhouse, 1995, p. 886) may not only be occasioned by ill health but also complicate the recovery of health and the maintenance of wellness. Unfortunately, spiritual distress is frequently misdiagnosed as inadequate coping, powerlessness, fearfulness, or emotional disturbance, and often mistreated with tranquilizers, reassurance, and advice. Parish nurses and congregational clergy can make major contributions to health care institutions by promoting recognition of and attention to spiritual distress.

Chaplains can also address the threefold etiology of spiritual distress: separation from religious ties, religious conflict or ethical dilemma regarding treatment, and/or the challenge of intense suffering (Kim, McFarland, and McLane, 1995, p. 78).

Spiritual Distress Related to Separation from Religious Ties

Spiritual distress may be precipitated by separation from the support provided by religious rituals and the communities of faith. Whether confined in a health care facility because of a traumatic injury or homebound due to chronic illness, individuals in ill health are frequently distressed by the loss of the religious elements in their lives that would normally reinforce their spiritual health and promote their general well-being. By providing and/or facilitating the provision of the "means of grace" (e.g., prayer, sacraments, religious literature) and contact with the faith community (e.g., visits from the individual's own clergy or by the chaplain), the chaplaincy service seeks to reduce the spiritual distress that can accompany the isolation of ill health. In the unfamiliar and distressing environment of the health care facility, "worship and prayer are a bridge to a more familiar, comfortable and reassuring world" (Watterson, 1997, p. 123).

Since chaplains are part of the medical care team and well acquainted with the peculiar world of the facility, they may be able to help the community clergy or other religious representatives to connect with and support individuals from their faith communities. Chaplains can advocate for the person and the faith community in their interactions with the health care system, providing aid simply by helping others find the right room, complying with isolation procedures, and negotiating time for sacraments or facilitating the sharing of information.

In addition, since the only empirical research available strongly suggests that we "cannot count on community religious caregivers, whether clergy or lay, to visit most or even a majority of the patients" (VandeCreek and Gibson, 1997, p. 413), the chaplain fills an important gap for many patients. This is particularly true when patients are geographically removed from their home worshiping community, "fallen away" from the practice of their faith, estranged from their congregation, or neglected by their clergy or congregation.

Pastoral care personnel have always had anecdotal evidence that such spiritual support improves health outcomes and also increases patient and family satisfaction. Empirical research has now clearly verified the practical benefits of spiritual support.[2] It is, however, important to remember that "the value of prayers or spiritual rituals to the believer is not affected by whether or not they can be scientifically 'proved' to be beneficial" (Carpenito, Mondoux, and Waterhouse, 1995, p. 888). Attention to a patient's religious needs and the provision of spiritual support are significant factors in caring for the person's total well-being within health care facilities:

> Spirituality/religion is a significant and honorable reality in the lives of many people. Under some circumstances spiritual con-

siderations can become more important than even physical survival. Pastoral care professionals can testify to this reality, but some . . . within the larger community of clinical professionals have perhaps forgotten that spiritual and religious realities need to be taken just as seriously as physical, psychological, social, and economic ones. (Buryska, 1999, p. 96)

Nevertheless, standards for hospital care recognize that "patients' psychosocial, spiritual, and cultural values affect how they respond to their care. [They mandate that] the hospital allows patients and their families to express their spiritual beliefs and cultural practices, as long as these do not harm others or interfere with treatment" (JCAHO, 1997, RI 8). "Many times it is the chaplain who ensures that everyone's traditions are respected, enabling everyone to practice his/her religion" (Watterson, 1997, p. 124). "The hospital chaplain, by training, is tolerant of all belief systems, and will assist patients and staff in having their particular spiritual needs met, either directly or by referral" (Wagner and Higdon, 1996, p. 16).

Spiritual Distress Related to Religious Conflict or Ethical Dilemma

The increasingly complex medical choices that confront people are often an additional and major source of spiritual distress. Decisions should be made on the basis of medical advice and the patient's values. When these values or their relation to the available choices are unclear, when they conflict with the values of family members, or when the opinion of the medical team conflicts with the values of the patient, severe spiritual distress and considerable practical confusion result. "It falls frequently to the . . . chaplain in a hospital to be the intersection of faith and science and to be a companion to the individual faced with seemingly conflicting values" (O'Brien, 1995, p. 280). The chaplain's familiarity with the language of values and ability to facilitate ethical discernment address these problems.[3]

Ethical consultations provided by chaplains often help individuals and groups to clarify their own values and arrive at a decision. In situations of conflict, chaplains can understand the patient's values or religious concerns, explain these to the family or the medical team, and advocate on the patient's behalf. Chaplains may also provide mediation or suggestions in order to facilitate the appropriate treatment. Chaplains "are often adept at conducting the most critical communication of all, the family conference about the decision at hand. For a family experiencing a standoff or impasse of decision-making, the pastoral care staff . . . are invaluable" (Poorman, 1994, p. 14). In this role, chaplains will not try to impose particular values but will help people discover, articulate, and examine their own convictions. Instead of trying to convert vulnerable people to a particular belief system, chaplains seek to encourage and strengthen the faith and the spiritual health already present. Finally, even when no specific ethical dilemma exists, just the experience of illness may cause patients to "be confronted with fundamental questions about their system of values and source of spiritual support. . . . Patients . . . confront these ultimate issues and may need help in their search for something to believe in and to hope for" (Shafer, 1991, p. 42). The expertise of chaplains in facilitating ethical dialogues concerning dilemmas as well as their attention to values clarification and the language of meaning will increasingly be in demand because modern medical decision making grows ever more complex, the values in American society more diverse, and family relations increasingly complicated.

In addition to being available to individual patients, family members, and medical staff, chaplains are often part of the institution's ethics committee:

> Chaplains bring the expertise in spiritual, theological, ethical, and moral values to the multidisciplinary reflection and discourse concerning ethical issues, dilemmas, case studies and retrospective reviews. [They] . . . have the experience and training that relates to effective group process, an essential ingredient for effective ethical decision-making. (Guss and the Bioethics Committee of the College of Chaplains, 1992, p. 2)

Spiritual Distress Related to the Challenge of Suffering

Intense suffering may also cause spiritual distress. Suffering includes ongoing physical discomfort and/or emotional distress accompanied by a perception of powerlessness or hopelessness and/or a sense of exhaustion. "Suffering is a spiritual phenomenon, an event that strikes at the faith we can have in life" (Van Hooft, 1998, p. 14). This spiritual crisis is a subjective experience that is not easily measured, but it is nonetheless very real and must be treated appropriately. Chaplains attend to those who suffer. "Chaplains . . . can approach people in . . . pain by meeting them in their spiritual crisis, by validating and encouraging good medical and psychological care, and by offering the resources of spirituality in concert with other treatments" (Mandziuk, 1993, p. 47). Although medication may effectively relieve pain and relaxation techniques may significantly reduce anxiety, suffering must also be addressed directly and personally. Suffering involves a crisis of ultimate meaning and hope. Chaplains "view spiritual or existential suffering as the core of the experience of suffering" (Handzo, 1996, p. 46). Chaplains are specifically trained to receive the concerns and emotions (including the rage!) that surround suffering, to be with the individual or family in the depth of despair, to speak to the deep questions, and to provide guidance and encouragement in the search for adequate understanding and comfort.

Suffering may be unavoidable, but it is not insurmountable, and chaplains are a crucial resource for helping people confront it. "Chaplains offer people alternatives to beliefs that cause suffering and help people strengthen beliefs that ward off distress" (Handzo, 1996, p. 45). This is especially true when suffering cannot be fully relieved. Inevitably, despite our best efforts, medicine, philosophy, pills, and prayers ultimately fail to eliminate every moment of personal pain or mortal angst. In these times "suffering is to be borne. There is nothing more to it" (Van Hooft, 1998, p. 19). During these times, chaplains are companions in the experience of suffering. Indeed, their capacity to accept pain and to remain fully present to people in distress may be the hallmark of pastoral care. This, as much as any prayer or pronouncement, may be the most articulate expression of the compassion of God and the strength of faith. This is vitally important because "in looking at our American culture . . . we see the forces of denial operating on a vast and pervasive scale, wanting to eliminate limitation, ignore dependency, and sweep out of sight whatever is or reflects pain and suffering in the human condition" (Gatti, 1975, p. 52). Chaplains can assist people as they face painful realities.

ADDITIONAL SERVICES OF CHAPLAINS

In conjunction with their focus on the spiritual health of the patients they serve, chaplains provide several additional services within health care systems. These include crisis intervention, communication enhancement and conflict resolution, discernment and referral, specialized and supplemental counseling, and promotion of spirit and values. Although each of these functions can be, and sometimes is, provided by other professions, pastoral care has a particular ability to deliver each of these services effectively.

Crisis Intervention

Crisis intervention is quite effectively provided by chaplains. Clergy, including chaplains, "have something nobody else has: the psychological and social right to take pastoral initiative in calling, visiting, and making contact" (Pruyser, 1972, p. 8). "This . . . inherent permission to take initiative with people without first being asked to help . . . may or may not be welcomed, but taking initiative is role-appropriate" (Wagner and Higdon, 1996, p. 19). Some people react to this initiative with anxiety, distrust, or hostility, generally because they are unfamiliar with the role of chaplains. They assume that the presence of the chaplain indicates that death is inevitable. Others suspect that this pious person will attempt to convert them to a particular religious persuasion, or at least make them feel guilty about their failings. Some people are uncomfortable with anyone not of their own faith. Occasionally, the pain of past or perceived misconduct by clergy is projected onto chaplains. Chaplains are trained to be sensitive to these reactions and are often able gently to overcome them. They clarify that their presence does not necessarily mean hopelessness. Chaplains also clearly affirm that, while they are open and honest about their own faith, they are committed to a code of ethics "which forbids proselytizing of persons under care in health care institutions" (Guss and the Bioethics Committee of the College of Chaplains, 1992, p. 1).[4] In addition, chaplains are trained to receive the suspicions and hostility of others nondefensively. They can help people process negative reactions to clergy and to resolve these concerns and feelings. The chaplain's continued availability and expression of genuine concern are often all that is needed to forge a working connection even with resistive people in the health care setting.

Using this pastoral initiative and access, chaplains intervene in crisis situations and provide a nonanxious presence to calm and comfort individuals in distress. Chaplains use their skill in pastoral attending (unconditional positive regard, active listening, empathy, congruence, and reflective clarification) in crisis situations.

As the word implies, pastoral care is "shepherding" (Hiltner, 1959, 1963). Chaplains guide and comfort vulnerable people through crisis. They enable people in crisis (e.g., parents arriving at the emergency department to learn of their child's accidental death, family members awaiting the outcome of resuscitation efforts, a patient receiving a terminal diagnosis) to gain perspective on the situation, mobilize their resources for coping, and, thus, find some realistic sense of order and control in the midst of chaos and perceived helplessness. Chaplains may also allow people in crisis to "lose it" for a time, by providing them the opportunity, and possibly even encouragement, to "act out" and release their emotions in relative safety.

Pastoral care interventions do not eliminate the crisis event, but the presence and activity of chaplains empower people in crisis to handle the ordeal. In addition, chaplains are able to provide spiritual support (e.g., scripture, prayer) and to address questions of meaning and hope (existential and theological concerns). "After the dialogue begins and initial rapport has been established, inevitably the ultimate questions [are] asked. . . . It is important to hear these questions, to which there are often no reasonable answers, [and] the feelings behind the questions need to be explored" (Gillman et al., 1996, pp. 15-16). In times of crisis, and especially in the presence of death, chaplains are widely recognized as having the right and the ability to understand and to respond, to listen and to speak. In the often traumatic world of health care, such services are crucial.

Obviously community clergy who have an ongoing supportive relationship with individuals and the family members involved are the best providers of crisis intervention. In some cases, chaplains contact a person's own clergy and then serve as a liaison with the medical team. Many times, however, there is no relationship with a clergy. Even when clergy are identified, their busy schedules may make them unavailable at the time of a sudden and unexpected crisis. In such cases, the availability of chaplains is particularly valuable.

Communication Enhancement and Conflict Resolution

The specialized and complex world of modern medicine is often frightening and bewildering to the general public. Information is not easily conveyed or assimilated. The stress of ill health and critical decision making may impair cognitive processing and find expression in displaced anger. Impaired communication and uncontained conflict are common, severely compromising medical efforts to be helpful. Chaplains often enhance communication and manage conflict.

Chaplains, similar to other clergy, can often help medical personnel translate their complex, specialized, and technical data and their opinions into language that patients and family members understand. At the same time, chaplains can help patients and families convey their inchoate understanding, their questions, and their hopes and fears to the medical team. Chaplains bring the additional valuable resources of familiarity with cultural diversity, experience in multicultural conversations, and ease in ecumenical situations.

Resolving conflict is also a particular calling of the clergy. Chaplains are often viewed as uniquely credible, fair, and nonthreatening in the midst of conflict, and with authority to advance resolution. Conflict resolution and "reconciliation [proceed] frequently through acts of convening, in which the clergy [or chaplain] may assume active group leadership, facilitate dialogue, play the role of mediator and arbiter, or merely enable human encounters by making arrangements for them" (Pruyser, 1972, p. 11).

The work of the chaplaincy service in enhancing communication and managing conflict helps save time, effort, difficulty, apprehension, and heartache.[5] Chaplains may be able to act as liaison for the parish nurse or community clergy. Such efforts may include persuading hospital personnel, including physicians, to communicate with the parish nurse, encouraging staff nurses to respect the congregational clergy's visits, or "refereeing" a family disagreement.

Discernment and Referral

Chaplains may provide clarification, share understanding, or recommend action in unusual or difficult patient situations. This discernment and referral service is often provided when a pastoral care referral is made due to a situation similar to spiritual distress (e.g., ineffective coping, diversional activity deficit, fear, noncompliance, self-esteem disturbance, social isolation, risk for violence, pain.)[6] Chaplains may use their privilege of pastoral access and their skill in pastoral attending to explore difficulties and resolve uncertainties. The chaplain is often able to recognize "the presence of one or more specific psychological or behavioral factors that adversely affect a general medical condition" (American Psychiatric Association [APA], 1994, p. 675).[7] With an understanding of the problem from the perspective of the people involved, chaplains are able to use their knowledge of available resources to suggest referrals for those who receive health care services. They are "trusted as referral channels and triage agents whose advice is appreciated when the question is, 'Where can I get help?' " (Pruyser, 1976, p. 45). Chaplains may also aid the physician in discussions about complementary or alternative treatments that patients often seek. Consultation among chaplains, parish nurses, and community clergy can be helpful for all three professionals.

Specialized and Supplemental Counseling

In addition, individual chaplains often have particular expertise to offer. Their specialized and supplemental counseling may focus on such disparate areas as domestic violence, mental illness, or employee assistance. Two very common examples are grief work and substance abuse treatment.

Grief is a distressing, natural process of responding to actual or anticipated loss and is subject to complications.[8] "The growing body of knowledge illustrate[s] that survivors [are] at higher risk for both morbidity and mortality" (Wolfelt, 1988, p. 83). Research on traumatically bereaved parents indicates that

> religious beliefs of the family and the religious support available were major determinants in outcome. . . . The recognition of religion's importance in the outcome of the grieving process

makes it ever more important that we involve the chaplain service early and thoroughly . . . in the management of all our critically ill patients. (Krizek, 1995, p. 308)

Chaplains are especially familiar with the difficult process of grieving, and they often provide counseling to individuals and families in order to foster its healthy resolution. Lament and memorial are inherently spiritual, and chaplains have expertise in the sacred language and rituals of mourning. As with crisis intervention, chaplains are particularly able to aid grieving people and to guide, comfort, and "bless" them in the task they face. Chaplains frequently meet with people in the initial, acute phase of grief reaction or anticipatory grieving within the health care setting (e.g., death, amputation, transition from independent living to a nursing home, loss of standard means of employment or income). Often called upon to assist with the "life review" that many terminal patients undertake, chaplains address the spiritual concerns of those facing death. They may also provide ongoing counseling throughout the grief process on an outpatient basis.

Recovery from substance abuse, with its radical change in lifestyle, commitments, and thinking, has many parallels with religious conversion. Alcoholics Anonymous has its roots in the religious disciplines. Because of these connections with spirituality, chaplains have a natural understanding of the dynamics involved and can support the individual and family in the process of recovery. For those individuals whose recovery involves an actual religious conversion or a revived sense of spirituality, chaplains may provide encouragement and insight into this new dimension of life, as well as referral to a faith community and clergy. Chaplains are frequently involved in helping people with the confessional fifth step of a twelve-step program. Chaplains often help with triage and referral for those seeking help with substance abuse, and many have special training and certification as addiction counselors as well.

Promotion of Spirit and Values

"In a medical center, ritual and discussions about hope or suffering apply equally to staff and patients. Chaplains, in caring for the human spirit, minister to the health care team members, ever reminding us of

God's presence" (Handzo, 1996, p. 47). Not only are chaplains available to health care staff for the regular services of pastoral care, they may also be able to provide extra service to their co-workers, including parish nurses and parish clergy, in the promotion of spirit and values. After particularly stressful events, chaplains may provide formal or informal critical incident stress debriefing for those involved. Chaplains are often involved in referring employees who are in need to the appropriate resources within the institution (e.g., an employee assistance program, financial crisis funds, emergency leave) or in the community (e.g., family counseling, social service agencies). Their regular assistance in stress management and in validating and encouraging individuals is particularly important in the strained and stressful workplace that is becoming more and more the norm in health care. In our present era of downsizing, chaplains also assist staff in managing the stress of job insecurity.

The contemporary environment of health care is particularly conducive to moral distress. "Moral distress arises when one knows the right thing to do, but institutional constraints make it nearly impossible to pursue the right course of action" (A. Jameton, quoted in Wilkinson, 1987/1988, p. 16). This experience is not only personally painful, but it can also have a negative impact on patient care (Wilkinson, 1987/1988). Chaplains are often able to help health care professionals to recognize moral distress and to choose appropriate coping strategies.

Chaplains often gently remind health care professionals of the values that undergird their work.[9] Whereas politicians and investors may see health care as a commodity that is marketed by an industry in an economic environment, chaplains encourage health care providers to recognize that the work of healing is a ministry, and to remember the ideals that motivated them to dedicate themselves to this vocation. Chaplains proclaim, in word and deed, by argument and encouragement, that, while the delivery and funding of health care is always changing, our mission as health care providers remains ever constant:

> Chaplains often find it difficult to play the prophet, to criticize the system of which they are a very integral part. To be a prophet in a system upon which you depend for your livelihood is difficult and requires prophetic courage. Many times the truth is spo-

ken not in words but in deeds which lead the institution where it would go. (Watterson, 1997, p. 125)

THE PROFESSION OF PASTORAL CARE

Chaplains are not merely peculiarly spiritual and somewhat gifted amateurs in the field of human service. Pastoral care is not something that just anyone with good intentions and a sincere faith is able to provide; it requires professional training in the first principles of spiritual reality, theological understanding, religious practice, faith development, and emotional process. "Chaplains have moved far beyond the days of addressing purely denominational and sacramental concerns or simply offering a friendly visit" (Mandziuk, 1994, p. 376).

Chaplains, "like all other professional workers, possess a body of theoretical and practical knowledge that is uniquely their own, evolved over years of practice by themselves and their forebears" (Pruyser, 1976, p. 10). Certification for work in pastoral care is provided by several different professional organizations with clear requirements for training and high standards of ethical practice.[10] Formal training usually includes undergraduate liberal arts and graduate pastoral and theological education. "While not stridently denominational, chaplains remain true to their religious traditions" (Watterson, 1997, p. 125). Most chaplains are either commissioned or ordained and they maintain ongoing accountability to a faith community and an ecclesiastical authority. "Many chaplains have served in local congregations prior to their service in a medical center" (Handzo, 1996, p. 46). In addition, chaplains ought to have specialized training through intensive clinical residencies in medical or psychiatric facilities (called clinical pastoral education [CPE]). This experience orients the chaplain-in-training to the health care environment and the disciplines of other health care professionals, hones the skills of pastoral care, and addresses the individual's personal strengths and challenges. Most chaplains have become familiar "with psychological and psychiatric knowledge, in the conviction that theoretical constructs and skills from these disciplines can make important contributions to enhancing the efficacy of pastoral work" (Pruyser, 1972, p. 5). Many chaplains have additional knowledge of ethics, education, or social work and experience in counseling, spiritual direction, or administration.

Chaplains and Congregational Ministers

Thus, a community "minister is usually a 'generalist,' whereas the hospital chaplain is a 'specialist'" (Wagner and Higdon, 1996, p. 16). Chaplains are usually more adept in ecumenical situations and more familiar with psychodynamics that occur in the health care milieu than local clergy. At the same time, chaplains are much less familiar with the people they meet than are congregational ministers. When interacting with people, chaplains are likely to focus on the particular situation in which they find themselves and the specific issues that arise from those circumstances; the congregational minister may be more able to speak to the larger context of the individual's life history and community of faith. Oddly enough, some people feel greater freedom sharing intimate vulnerabilities with the chaplain, who is a relative stranger, than with their own clergy, with whom they have a richer but more complex and complicated relationship. Since chaplains are not in a position of official responsibility for promoting a specific religious dogma, their attention to what is spiritual may be more likely to transcend the boundaries of what is usually considered "religious." Chaplains will generally spend less time performing specific religious rituals and more time actively listening to patients and their families. Thus, chaplains are often able to address the spiritual need of individuals who profess a different faith, as well as those who may be indifferent or even hostile to formal religious institutions.

Chaplains and Parish Nurses

The parish nurse is often the one person outside the patient's own family who is most extensively and intimately involved in the individual's health care. Nurses usually take a holistic approach to people and are thus quite naturally involved in attending to the spiritual aspects of individuals and families. "Meeting spiritual needs is and always has been part of the nursing role" (Carson, 1989, p. 155). The nurse is most likely to listen and pay attention to the patient. "Many times the client expresses heartfelt spiritual needs" (Carson, 1989, p. 154) to the nurse. It should be noted, however, that "nursing curricula focus on biopsychosocial needs, with little if any solid content devoted to the spiritual dimension. . . . Nurses who have never received instruction in this area may recognize its importance but are professionally uncomfortable when intervening" (Carson, 1989, p. 154).[11] Nevertheless, a nurse who has chosen parish nursing over other, probably more prestigious and profitable, opportunities in the profession has a strong religious commitment and a mature faith. This nurse will most likely provide the compassionate presence and empathetic listening that the patients need most of all. The parish nurse may also be well able to pray with the patient, discuss matters of belief, and enlist other members of the faith community in support of the patient. Collaboration with the congregational minister and health care chaplains is appropriate for the parish nurse.

CONCLUSION

Some chaplains are hired and paid by religious or independent agencies that then contract with the health care institution to provide pastoral care services. Nevertheless, it is recommended that

> the chaplain in the general hospital [or other health care institution] . . . shall be responsible to someone in the . . . hospital regardless of who appoints him and pays his salary . . . [because] the chaplain is a member of the hospital team, along with the nurse, the dietitian, the social worker, the occupational therapist . . . the physician. . . . Only as he can adjust to this working relationship has he any place in the hospital of today, regardless of what may have been true in the past. (Dicks, 1996/1940, p. 2)

"Doctors and medical administrators familiar with chaplaincy programs praise . . . their effectiveness in helping people cope with, if not recover from, catastrophic illness and in broadening the medical team's ability to treat the whole person" (Gonzalez, 1994, p. B1). Because outcomes are enhanced, pastoral care is increasingly being integrated into clinical pathways (Hudson, 1996). Most chaplains are eager to work collaboratively and will continue to share their special gifts with the entire health care team, including the parish nurse and the congregational minister.

NOTES

1. The chaplain's concern could be coded from the *Diagnostic and Statistical Manual of Mental Disorders,* Fourth Edition (DSM-IV) as "V62.89 Religious or Spiritual Problem" (American Psychiatric Association [APA], 1994, p. 685).

2. Extensive information of collected results and ongoing research may be obtained from the National Institute for Healthcare Research, Suite 908, 6110 Executive Blvd., Rockville, MD 20852, <www.nihr.org>. See also Marwick, 1995, and Wallis, 1996.

3. Some of the situations addressed here could be categorized as DSM-IV "V15.81 Noncompliance With Treatment" (APA, 1994, p. 683).

4. From the Code of Ethics of the Association of Professional Chaplains (http://www.professionalchaplains.org/aboutapc/code.htm/): "Members treat all persons with respect, recognizing the dignity and worth of each individual. Members celebrate diversity and serve all persons regardless of religion, race, ethnicity, sexual orientation, age, disability, or gender. Members affirm the spiritual and religious freedom of all persons and refrain from proselytizing."

5. The DSM-IV code for these circumstances is "V61.9 Relational Problem Related to a Mental Disorder or General Medical Condition" (APA, 1994, p. 681).

6. See Gordon, 1982, or other manuals of nursing diagnosis.

7. The applicable "DSM- IV code is 316 Psychological Factor Affecting Medical Condition." (APA, 1994, p. 678). Another possibly applicable code is "307.89 Pain Disorder Associated With Both Psychological Factors and a General Medical Condition" (APA, 1994, p. 458).

8. This service may be correlated with the condition coded as DSM-IV "V62.82 Bereavement" (APA, 1994, p. 684).

9. This may or may not be within the formal scope of the pastoral care department. In my own health care system there is an executive, a religious sister from the sponsoring order, who is responsible for articulating our mission and values and overseeing their implementation. In other systems it may be the CEO who provides the vision, or the marketing department that articulates the virtues of the system. Regardless, the chaplain will speak to mission and values.

10. The following organizations may be contacted for further information: Association of Professional Chaplains (recently formed by the merger of the College of Chaplains and the Association of Mental Health Clergy), 1701 E. Woodfield Rd., Schaumburg, IL 60173, <www.professionalchaplains.org>; National Association of Catholic Chaplains, P.O. Box 07473, Milwaukee, WI 53207, <www.nacc.org>; Association for Death Education and Counseling, 638 Prospect Ave., Hartford, CT 06105, <www.adec.org>; American Association of Pastoral Counselors, 9504a Lee Hgwy, Fairfax, VA 22031, <www.aapc.org>; Association for Clinical Pastoral Education, 1549 Clairmont Rd., Decatur, GA 30033, <www.acpe.edu>.

11. Stronger words have been used of physicians: "Many of us involved in the medical profession have not been taught about religion, and this most important part of life, for most people, is not a subject that many of us feel equipped to approach and, therefore, tend to ignore as either 'not important' or 'not important to what we do!' " (Krizek, 1995, p. 308). Nevertheless, it should be noted that the medical com-

munity, along with the general public, has recently showed a renewed interest in the positive health effects of religion and spirituality (Marwick, 1995; Wallis, 1996). In fact, a recent study of family physicians found that "more than 80 percent of the physicians reported that they refer or recommend their patients to clergy and pastoral care providers . . . [and concluded that] most family physicians accept clergy and pastoral professionals in the care of their patients. In medical settings, the providers of religious and spiritual interventions have a larger and more expanded role than previously reported" (Daaleman and Frey, 1998, p. 548).

REFERENCES

American Psychiatric Association [APA] (1994). *Diagnostic and statistical manual of mental disorders,* Fourth edition. Washington, DC: American Psychiatric Association, pp. 458-462, 675-678, 680-685.

Buryska, J. (1999). Final say—A pastoral voice in the health care wilderness. *Health Progress, 80*(2), 96.

Carpenito, L., Mondoux, L., and Waterhouse, J. (1995). Spiritual distress. In L. Carpenito (ed.), *Nursing diagnosis: Application to clinical practice.* New York: J.B. Lippincott, pp. 886-903.

Carson, V. (1989). Spirituality and the nursing process. In V. Carson (ed.), *Spiritual dimensions of nursing practice.* Philadelphia, PA: W.B. Saunders, pp. 150-179.

Daaleman, T. and Frey, B. (1998). Prevalence and patterns of physician referral to clergy and pastoral care providers. *Archives of Family Medicine, 7,* 548-553.

Dicks, R. (1996/1940). The work of the chaplain in a general hospital. *The Caregiver Journal, 12,* 2-5. Reprinted from *American Protestant Hospital Association Bulletin, 4,* 1-4.

Gatti, D. (1975). The hospital chaplain and his ministry. *AMHC Forum, 27,* 51-55.

Gillman, J., Gable-Rodriquez, J., Sutherland, M., and Whitacre, J. (1996). Pastoral care in a critical care setting. *Critical Care Nursing Quarterly, 19,* 10-20.

Gonzalez, D. (1994). Tending the spirit as well as the body. *The New York Times,* September 7, B1-B2.

Gordon, M. (1982). *Manual of nursing diagnosis.* New York: McGraw-Hill, p. 226.

Guss, V. and the Bioethics Committee of the College of Chaplains (1992). Guidelines for the chaplain's role in bioethics. Paper circulated to *Association of Professional Chaplains* members.

Handzo, G. (1996). Chaplaincy: A continuum of caring. *Oncology, 10,* 45-47.

Hiltner, S. (1959). *The christian shepard.* Nashville, TN: Abingdon Press.

Hiltner, S. (1963). *Preface to pastoral theology.* Nashville, TN: Abingdon Press.

Hudson, T. (1996). Measuring the results of faith. *Hospitals and Health Networks, 70,* 22-28.

Joint Commission on Accreditation of Healthcare Organizations (1997). *Comprehensive accreditation manual for hospitals.* RI 1-21.

Kim, M., McFarland, G., and McLane, A. (1995). *Pocket guide to nursing diagnoses.* St. Louis, MO: Mosby, pp. 78-79, 420-424.

Krizek, T. (1995). Editorial. *The Journal of Trauma: Injury, Infection, and Critical Care, 39,* 303-308.

Larson, D., Swyers, J., and McCullough, M. (eds.) (1998). *Scientific research on spirituality and health: A consensus report.* Rockville, MD: National Institute for Healthcare Research.

Levin, J. and Larson, D. (1997). Religion and spirituality in medicine: Research and education. *Journal of the American Medical Association, 278,* 792-793.

Mandziuk, P. (1993). Easing chronic pain with spiritual resources. *Journal of Religion and Health, 32,* 47-54.

Mandziuk, P. (1994). The doctor-chaplain relationship. *Western Journal of Medicine, 160,* 376-377.

Marwick, C. (1995). Should physicians prescribe prayer for health? Spiritual aspects of well-being considered. *Journal of the American Medical Association, 273,* 1561-1562.

O'Brien, W. (1995). Dialogue between faith and science: The role of the hospital chaplain. *Journal of Clinical Ethics, 6,* 280-284.

Poorman, M. (1994). The family in end-of-life decisions. *America, 171,* 12-15.

Pruyser, P. (1972). The use and neglect of pastoral resources. *Pastoral Psychology, 23,* 5-17.

Pruyser, P. (1976). *The minister as diagnostician.* Philadelphia, PA: Westminster Press.

Shafer, J. (1991). Spiritual distress and critical illness. *Critical Care Nurse, 11,* 42-45.

Van Hooft, S. (1998). The meaning of suffering. *Hastings Center Report, 28,* 13-19.

VandeCreek, L. and Gibson, S. (1997). Religious support from parish clergy for hospitalized parishioners: Availability, evaluation, implications. *The Journal of Pastoral Care, 51,* 403-414.

Wagner, J. and Higdon, T. (1996). Spiritual issues and bioethics in the intensive care unit: The role of the chaplain. *Critical Care Clinics, 12,* 15-27.

Wallis, C. (1996). Faith and healing. *Time,* June 24, 58-64.

Watterson, J. (1997). Tell it to the chaplain. *Medicine and Health/Rhode Island, 80,* 123-125.

Wilkinson, J. (1987/1988). Moral distress in nursing practice: Experience and effect. *Nursing Forum, 23,* 16-29.

Wolfelt, A. (1988). *Death and grief: A guide for clergy.* Muncie, IN: Accelerated Development Publishing.

SECTION II:
RELIGIOUS AND THEOLOGICAL
CONSIDERATIONS

Chapter 3

Toward a Christian Theology of Nursing

Judith Allen Shelly

A HISTORY OF NURSING AND THE CHURCH

Martha, a former nursing educator with a PhD in nursing, exclaimed in wonder, "I quit my high-paying teaching job to become a parish nurse—*this* is what I came into nursing to be!" She seems typical of many parish nurses. Most are mature, competent nurses with strong faith commitment and a vision for serving God through nursing.

Jesus' teaching and example of caring for the sick created a Christian worldview that in turn gave birth to nursing. The current parish nurse movement has grown out of this vision for nursing as a ministry of the Christian church. The concepts of God, the person, the church, the environment, health, and the role of parish nursing as a ministry are uniquely Christian.

My own story mirrors this pattern. I entered nursing inspired by Jesus' example and teaching. I wanted to serve God by caring for the sick. From the beginning, I realized that a nursing career was no easy commitment, and that nursing was a deeply spiritual endeavor. My first patient had tried to commit suicide by shooting himself in the mouth. Instead, he lost half his face, including one eye, his nose, and all but a tiny hole for a mouth. He needed more than physical care—care that I did not know how to provide at the time. As my career developed, patients frequently asked me to pray for them. Others asked, "Why did God allow this to happen to me?" Finally, I went to seminary, seeking answers and ministry skills.

An earlier version of these materials was presented at the Thirteenth Annual Granger Westberg Symposium, Itasca, Illinois, September 16, 1999.

During my seminary experience, I took one unit of clinical pastoral education, then completed my fieldwork as a hospital chaplain in the same hospital where I worked as a nurse on weekends. As I cared for patients in both roles (sometimes the same patients), a fascinating pattern became evident. When I cared for patients as a nurse, they would frequently tell me their deepest concerns and ask me to pray for them. When I offered to pray for them (even without being asked), they never refused. However, when I visited as a chaplain, patients put on their best facade of holiness and respectability. They seldom confessed their fears and doubts, and they sometimes told me they did not need my prayers.

One of my most fascinating chaplain experiences resulted from a previous experience with a patient as a nurse. I first met Joe Levi when he was admitted to hospital with prostate cancer. After surgery, he experienced intractable pain. As a nurse, I gave him all the analgesics his physician would allow and irrigated his urinary catheter to remove any blood clots, but he still writhed in agony. Finally, I said that all I could do was pray. He desperately accepted my offer. I prayed to the "God of Abraham, Isaac, and Jacob," thanking him for his faithfulness to his people and asking for his healing hand to rest upon Joe. Afterward, Joe promptly fell asleep, obviously relieved of pain, but when he awoke he wanted to talk. He poured out his anger at God for allowing his relatives to be tortured or killed in the Holocaust and told me his family history. He was afraid God would not help him anymore because of his anger. I read him a psalm in which the psalmist cried out in anger to God, but at the end was reminded of God's faithfulness. Joe asked for a Bible, so I gave him my pocket nurses' New Testament and Psalms, explaining that I did not have a Jewish Bible.

Several months later, while making my rounds as a chaplain, Joe came running out of the family waiting room next to the operating room. He grabbed my arm, pulling me into the waiting room toward a large gathering of crying people, announcing, "This nurse prays!" I am sure his family members were bewildered as I stood there in street clothes wearing a badge that clearly identified me as a chaplain. Then Joe introduced me as his nurse during his previous hospitalization, and he explained to me that his daughter was in surgery for suspected cancer of the gall bladder. He insisted we all stand and hold hands while I prayed for his daughter. I complied; soon afterward the surgeon told them that no cancer was evident.

The experience with Joe only confirmed my desire to be a nurse. If a rabbi or a chaplain had visited Joe during his hospitalization, I seriously doubt that he would have expressed his anger toward God. However, as a nurse, I had already crossed the intimacy barrier. After all, I had just given him a belladonna and opium suppository and irrigated his urinary catheter. He probably figured he had no privacy to lose by baring his soul. Nursing provided a profound entry into the spiritual dimension of those in my care.

Twenty years later, after a career of teaching and writing about spiritual care in nursing, I entered parish nursing through the back door. As a doctoral student of ministry, I was developing a curriculum in health ministries for my dissertation and needed a clinical position for the program outcome. Parish nursing seemed logical and I volunteered as a parish nurse in my congregation. Again, I discovered all that I had entered nursing to be and do.

Another experience opened my eyes to the unique connection between nursing and faith. As part of a church bazaar, the volunteer parish nurses in my congregation offered a health fair. I assisted a nurse and several technicians from our local hospital with free blood glucose and cholesterol screening. Several participating church members told us that they had never had their blood checked for anything in the past. They listened intently to our health teaching and continued to return for monthly blood pressure screening and occasional consultations about health concerns. Phil, an elderly diabetic in my Sunday school class, came to have his blood checked after a bit of friendly small talk. His blood sugar was dangerously high, so we called his physician, who agreed to meet him at the emergency room (where it was even higher). Afterward, I talked with him about following his diet and regularly taking his medication. Later, his wife confided, "He never would listen to the doctor, but he's taking what you say seriously." He has now outlived his wife.

The nurse from our local hospital who was part of the health fair has since remarked several times about the great value of church-based health care. She observed, "They came to the screening because they trusted you. With that trust they overcame their fear." That trust continues to build, and I see people living healthier lives because I am a parish nurse.

My own experience resonates with that of other parish nurses. We realize anew that faith is integral to good health and that nursing naturally belongs in the church.

The current parish nurse movement is really not new. The Christian church significantly influenced nursing and health care from the very beginning. Although some forms of health care were provided in ancient cultures, nurse historian Patricia Donahue (1996) states, "The history of nursing first becomes continuous with the beginning of Christianity" (p. 93). Dolan, Fitzpatrick, and Herrmann (1983) state:

> The teachings and example of *Jesus Christ* had a profound influence on the emergence of gifted nurse leadership as well as on the expansion of the role of nurses. Christ stressed the need to love God and one's neighbor. The first organized group of nurses was established as a direct response to His example and challenge. (p. 43)

This movement began when the first-century Christians began to teach that all persons were ministers who were to care for the poor, the sick, and the disenfranchised as described in the New Testament (Matthew 25:31-46, Hebrews 13:1-3, James 1:27, 1 Peter 2:9). For instance, Clark (1983) quotes St. Jerome who wrote of the early deaconess, Fabiola:

> And at first [Fabiola] established a hospital, into which she gathered the sick off the streets, where she might restore the limbs of the wretched that were wasted with weakness and starvation. . . . How often did she wash the corruption and bloody pus from wounds which some other man did not dare to glimpse? (pp. 182-183)

As the churches grew, the leaders appointed deacons to care for the needy within the congregations (Barnett, 1995). Eventually, more men and women were added to the roll of deacons and their designated responsibilities grew to include caring for the sick (Zersen, 1994). Dolan, Fitzpatrick, and Herrmann (1983) claim that Phoebe, the deacon mentioned in Romans 16:1-2, was the first visiting nurse. By the third century, organized groups of deaconesses were caring for the sick, the insane, and lepers in the community (Haazig, 1989).

In the fourth century, the church began establishing hospitals. Physicians often did not staff these hospitals because, during several periods, the early church did not condone the practice of medicine, viewing it as a pagan art (Bullough and Bullough, 1987). Nurse historians Dock and Stewart (1931) state:

> The age-old custom of hospitality . . . was practiced with religious fervor by the early Christians. . . . Their houses were opened wide to every afflicted applicant and, not satisfied with receiving needy ones, the deacons, men and women alike, went out to search and bring them in. The private homes of the deacons were turned into hospitals called diakonia, and the name deacon became synonymous with that of a director of hospital relief. (p. 51)

Nursing in the Middle Ages was centered in monasteries. Women who wanted to serve God and care for the sick joined together in monastic orders. By the late Middle Ages, the Hospitallers of St. John of Jerusalem, a military nursing order, built hospitals, one in Jerusalem and others along the route of the Crusades. Although the original intent was to care for Christian pilgrims, they also cared for Muslims, Jews, and crusaders (Carson, 1989).

The Renaissance through the eighteenth century brought a dark period in the history of nursing. As Catholic religious orders were disbanded or suppressed in Protestant countries, hospitals deteriorated. Nursing ceased to be a public role, moving out of the church and into the home. However, some religious orders in southern Europe continued to provide nursing care, including those established by St. Francis de Sales (1567-1662) and St. Vincent de Paul (1576-1669) (Carson, 1989). Care deteriorated, even among the religious orders, as nuns were not allowed to touch any part of the human body except the head and extremities, and they were often forced to work twenty-four-hour shifts (Dock and Stewart, 1931).

By the nineteenth century, except for a few orders of nuns, nursing was disorganized and corrupt. Dolan, Fitzpatrick, and Herrmann (1983) describe hospitals in Philadelphia in 1884:

Hospital patients were penniless folk, usually homeless and friendless. In most of the city hospitals, the nursing was done by inmates usually over 50 years old, many being 70 or 80. . . . There was practically no night nursing, except for the "night watchers" provided for women in childbirth and the dying. (p. 137)

Charles Dickens (1868) portrayed nineteenth-century nursing in the character of Sairey Gamp in his novel *Martin Chuzzlewit.* Dickens focused public attention on the nursing care being provided by alcoholics, prostitutes, and women who were uncaring and immoral. A self-seeking alcoholic, Gamp has become the symbol of nursing at its worst.

Reform again came through the work of the Christian church. Elizabeth Seton established the Widow's Society in New York to care for poor women in their homes. She later joined the Catholic Church and eventually established the Sisters of Charity at Emmitsburg, Maryland. Mother Mary Catherine McAuley founded the Sisters of Mercy who ministered among the poor and sick in Dublin, Ireland; eventually it spread to other countries, including the United States. Elizabeth Fry, an American Quaker in London began a campaign of prison reform that eventually developed into the Society of Protestant Sisters of Charity whose primary objective was to supply nurses for the sick of all classes in their homes (Carson, 1989).

Fry had a strong influence on a German Lutheran pastor, Theodor Fliedner, and his wife, Frederika. Seeing the pressing needs of the poor and the sick in their community, the Fliedners decided that the church must care for them. They turned a little garden house into a home for outcast girls and eventually organized a community of deaconesses to visit and nurse the sick in their homes. That experiment quickly grew into the Kaiserswerth Institute for the Training of Deaconesses, with a huge complex of buildings, including a hospital, and educational programs for nurses and teachers (Wentz, 1936).

About the same time, a young woman in England, Florence Nightingale, felt God calling her to future "service." She responded to that call by becoming a nurse, studying first at the Kaiserswerth Institute, then at Catholic hospitals in Paris. Nightingale went on to single-handedly reform nursing, bringing it back to its Christian roots and setting high educational and practice standards (Coakley, 1989).

However, her theological influence also set the stage for an ongoing struggle between those of her followers who wanted to be viewed as "professional" and those who understood nursing as a calling from God, a conflict Nightingale herself did not envision.

Nightingale dabbled in diverse philosophies and religions in her early years (Calabria and Macrae, 1994), but after she directed the nursing care of British soldiers in the Crimean War, her beliefs became more orthodox. It was in those later years that she began writing about nursing. Throughout her life, she seemed to see God and natural law as more or less the same. She had a deep, mystical relationship with God, whom she viewed as Absolute Perfection, Wisdom, and Love. She was overwhelmed with the love shown by Christ on the cross (Widerquist, 1995) but also deeply influenced by both Eastern and Western mysticism and by the theology of Friedrich Schleiermacher. However, Widerquist (1992) asserts that even when Nightingale received her call to good work, "It came to a young woman already prepared for the notion of working for God" (p. 108). Yet, to a great extent, she saw that service as a means of earning her own salvation.

During this time, churches in Europe and the United States began establishing hospitals with schools of nursing. William Passavant, a Lutheran pastor and pioneer in hospital development, visited Kaiserswerth and brought deaconesses to Pittsburgh, Pennsylvania, to staff his first hospital. The growing division between "professional nurse" and deaconess was already evident at this time. Passavant (1903) described the tension between Christian service and professionalism in an address given in 1899:

> The deaconess has a Biblical office, the nurse a worldly vocation. The one serves through love; the other for her support. In the one case we have an exercise of charity as wide in extent as the sufferings and misery of mankind; in the other, a usefulness circumscribed by the narrow circle of obedient help given to the physicians and surgeons. Above all, the deaconess cares for the body in order to reach the soul. She works for eternity. The trained nurse, like the man whose vocation brings him to the sick-bed, is as a rule, quite content to pass by unnoticed the possibilities of an eternal future in the demands of the present welfare of the patient. (p. 585)

One particular deaconess of this era, highlighted in a ninth-grade catechetical book, was Elizabeth Fedde. Sister Elizabeth studied nursing in Norway but traveled to New York at her own expense after receiving a letter from her brother-in-law in Brooklyn who described the desperate need for medical care of the Norwegian immigrants and seamen. At first she worked for a meager salary, which she supplemented by begging door-to-door. She formed a group called the Norwegian Relief Society that eventually grew into the Brooklyn Deaconess Hospital (now Fairview Hospital). Later, she was asked to establish a similar hospital in Minneapolis. She trained young women to be deaconess nurses and helped start the hospital that became Fairview Deaconess Hospital in Minneapolis (Burow, 1985).

The Tension Between Christian and Secular Nursing

Influential nursing leaders at the turn of the twentieth century railed against the idea of nursing as a religious calling for several reasons (Hamilton, 1994; Dock and Stewart, 1931). British empiricism encouraged disillusionment with the church and confidence in science. Most nurses in the religious orders and deaconess communities worked under oppressive conditions, resulting in chronic fatigue and a high mortality rate (Dock and Stewart, 1931). At the same time, the American social context included a strong sense of "progress" and an assumption that freedom and democracy would eventually create a pure, rational society. Rapid industrialization, however, had left society with a loss of community and large populations of disenfranchised poor. Upper-middle-class women, as keepers of the culture's mores and unable to hold paying jobs, became social reformers. Public health nursing arose out of these developments. Nurse historian Hamilton (1994) comments about these nurse reformers (inventors):

> Thus, both nursing and religion, if pursued compassionately, healed wounded minds, bodies, and spirits. Although the nurse inventors intended an unyielding boundary between religion and nursing, the kindred missions of religion and nursing rendered the boundary translucent. They envisioned that secular nursing would emulate the values of the religious sisters without accepting their rules, regulations, and cloistered life. Compas-

sion, once associated with God's authority, would, according to the nurse inventors, be replaced with compassion based on commitment to the authority of humanity and its social progress. (pp. 21-22)

Other nursing leaders during the same period insisted that the intimacy inherent in nursing practice required religious goodness, credulity, discipline, and obedience. Aikens, in a 1924 nursing ethics text, acknowledged religion, defined as "the relation which an individual fixes between his soul and his God" (pp. 51-52), as the basis for nursing ethics. Rebecca McNeill, RN, wrote in the *American Journal of Nursing* in 1910 that the "ideal nurse" must be a Christian (p. 393). Adding to the tension was the common practice of deaconess hospitals establishing schools of nursing based on the Nightingale system, so that, until the establishment of baccalaureate nursing programs, the two philosophies—service and professionalism—developed side by side.

While professional nursing grew in Western countries, the evangelical missionary movement also began. Early missionaries went to Asia and Africa, communicating the gospel primarily through education and health care. Florence Nightingale also sent out "missioners" to all English-speaking countries (Dock and Stewart, 1931, pp. 187-191). Although determined to be "secular," most drew their motivation from Christian faith and often worked through religious orders or mission hospitals. As missionary activity spread around the world, nursing worldwide could trace its roots to Florence Nightingale and a Christian worldview.

Nightingale's desire to make nursing a secular order has largely prevailed over the deaconess spirit of Christian service. The nursing profession today is primarily a secular one. The idea of nursing as *service* is scorned by many because it implies that nurses must be subservient. Although some church-related schools of nursing continue to exist, for the most part, nursing education today takes place in secular academic institutions. However, does faith continue to motivate and sustain Christian nurses today? Today's parish nurse movement is strong evidence that the idea of nursing as Christian service has not died.

HOW THEOLOGY INFORMS NURSING

Nursing practice today begins with a theoretical framework. Theories give meaning to observations and facts by placing them in an orderly system. Until recently, nursing was based on a theological perspective—it was one way to put the gospel into action. However, as nursing sought to gain professional recognition and respect, an effort to develop other theoretical frameworks began in the late 1950s. From 1950-1970, most nursing theories were based on a modern scientific worldview and gave rise to quantitative research in nursing. However, as researchers became dissatisfied with the inadequacy of science to measure the effects of holistic care, more recent theorists moved into a postmodern worldview, resulting in a rise in qualitative research. Neither of these worldviews is fully compatible with Christian belief nor with each other. Only a biblical theology fully accounts for both the physical and spiritual aspects of human existence, thus demonstrating the need for theological foundations.

Nursing theories are built upon four basic concepts: the person, the environment, health, and nursing. The way each of these concepts is defined influences the research questions, the interpretation of results, and the nature of nursing care. Historically, Christian faith was the original impetus for nursing and provided insight into each of these concepts. Undergirding our understanding of each concept is our understanding of the nature of God. Three worldviews shape these paradigms in today's nursing: modern, postmodern, and biblical. The biblical worldview specifically informs parish nursing practice.

Modernism

The modern worldview began with seventeenth-century philosopher René Descartes and his declaration *Cogito ergo sum* (I think, therefore I am). He advocated a mechanistic model of the universe and radical distinction between soul and body, opening the door to scientific inquiry and technological development. Descartes, while a faithful Roman Catholic, also insisted on making the existence of God subject to reason (Descartes, 1641/1969).

Modernism gave rise to a practical deism. Although the existence of God was accepted, God was viewed as a heavenly clockmaker who created the world, wound it up, and left it to run on its own, leaving

humans in charge. Truth became objective, measurable, and empiri-
cally discerned. Any supernatural intervention was considered mere
superstition and discounted. The individual person was seen as an
amazing complex machine that could be studied, improved, and fixed
when necessary. Health was considered the absence of disease, and
rapid advances in medicine and technology underscored that idea.
Vaccines, antibiotics, and other wonder drugs, along with new surgical techniques, extended life spans, and improved quality of life.
Spirituality and religious practice continued but were considered private matters that should not influence or interfere with public life.
"The research says" became the gold standard for truth in modernist
thinking. When we set out to prove through empirical research that
prayer "works" or that church attendance will lower your blood pressure, we draw on the modernist tradition.

The amazing benefits of technology and scientific medicine have
come with a price. The public reacted negatively to the coldness of
technology and began to fear the possibility of being kept alive indef-
initely while attached to tubes and wires. The limits of technology became evident as AIDS, drug-resistant tuberculosis, "killer strep," and
other new diseases arrived on the scene. Health care became exorbi-
tantly expensive. Feminism looked at modernism as a patriarchal system designed to control without respect for human spirituality or personal autonomy.

The nursing profession has become increasingly uncomfortable
with the modern worldview. Nurses have always sensed that a person
is much more than the physical body. While physical care has been an
essential aspect of nursing care, nurses have instinctively cared for
the spirit as well. It is no secret to a nurse that faith and health are integrally related. We have seen patients recover against all odds when
they sensed a higher purpose to their lives. We have also seen the
spirit go out of others when they gave up and died.

Postmodernism

More recently, nursing is moving into a new postmodern paradigm. A paradigm is a model, or a way of thinking and acting, a way
of viewing the world. Postmodernism began in the midtwentieth century with literary criticism that took issue with modernist dualism.
Postmodernism declares that no absolutes exist—everything is rela-

tive. It encourages multiculturalism, "political correctness," and a new tribalism. However, it also allows for spirituality to flourish—or, more accurately, for many spiritualities to appear.

Postmodernism is not one uniform worldview; as many worldviews as people exist. The assumption is that we each construct our own reality. In postmodernism, God can be almost anything you want and is often understood as energy. Many postmodernists credit Albert Einstein with making energy, and therefore God, relative. For example, James Gleick (1999), writing in *Time,* provides interesting commentary on Einstein's view of God:

> In embracing Einstein, our century took leave of a prior universe and an erstwhile God. The new versions were not so rigid and deterministic as the old Newtonian world. Einstein's God was no clockmaker, but he was the embodiment of reason in nature (subtle he is not). This God did not control our actions or even sit in judgment on them. . . . This God seemed rather kindly and absentminded, as a matter of fact. (p. 78)

More recently, the postmodern view of God has drifted into monism—believing that "all is one"—that nevertheless allows for the presence of other spiritual beings. Since this God/Energy is One with all things, I am God, you are God, and so are the animals, trees, streams, and rocks. This energy, sometimes called *chi, ki, prana,* or life force, can be manipulated by the mind and balanced through various healing modalities. Angels, spirit guides, and other forms of spiritual beings, including gods and goddesses, may be consulted and implored to assist with various alternative therapies.

Truth in the postmodern worldview is personally constructed. What is true for me, may not be true for you. There is no universal truth. Logical arguments and quantitative research findings hold little weight for postmodernists. If something feels like it works for me, then I will use it, even if no empirical evidence for its efficacy exists.

The postmodern environment is comprised of spiritual energy. The material world is seen as an illusion, and it can be moved around with the mind. No actual distinctions between people exist, nor clear boundaries to our bodies; only variations of intensity. The earth is viewed as a living organism, or as the goddess Gaia. Jean Watson

(1994), former president of the National League for Nursing, writes from a postmodern position when she asks:

> Can you consider a place that is not human-centered; where, instead, the human is decentered and takes this place in the context of a living cosmology, perhaps what I would call a living-caring cosmology that makes room for the Great Mother, the giver of life and creator of all? . . . [D]o we know that this is a turning by attunement, a harmonizing of the heavens and earth, an appeasement of the gods and goddesses of the universe? (pp. 30, 32)

Humans, in the postmodern worldview, are comprised of energy as well. The late Martha Rogers (1983), formerly head of the Division of Nursing at New York University, and mother of the new paradigm in nursing, defined the person as a unitary human being—an energy field that is an open system in continuous process with the environment. She acknowledged that this definition requires a new worldview.

Most advocates of postmodern thinking look to Eastern philosophy to explain how this human energy functions and can be manipulated for healing. They use traditional Chinese and Ayurvedic maps of meridians and chakras to locate these energy points; a quick search of the Internet yields hundreds, perhaps thousands, of similar approaches.

Nursing theorist and researcher Rosemarie Parse (1995) builds on this understanding of the person, stating:

> The human is: (1) coexisting while coconstituting rhythmical patterns with the universe, (2) an open being, freely choosing meaning in situations, bearing responsibility for decisions, (3) a living unity continuously coconstituting patterns in relating, and (4) transcending multidimensionally with the possibles. (pp. 5-6)

"Health" in the postmodern worldview can be whatever you—or your patient—want it to be. In Parse's (1995) theory, the concept of health has now evolved into "becoming." She no longer even uses the term *health*. "Becoming is: (1) a rhythmically coconstituting human-universe process, (2) the human's pattern of relating value priorities, (3) an intersubjective process of transcending with the possibles, and (4) human evolving" (p. 6). For nursing theorist Margaret Newman (Hensley et al., 1986), health is "expanding consciousness" (p. 371).

Postmodernist "health care" becomes a confusing blend of conventional and alternative (also called complementary) therapies, which may be contradictory or even counterproductive, but they are ultimately chosen by the health care recipient. We have moved away from the concept of *patient* to *client,* and more recently to *consumer,* each term bearing very different implications and increasing degrees of autonomy. Television and magazines advertise prescription drugs, assuming the consumer has more wisdom than the physician about the drugs in question. "Natural" and herbal remedies are marketed for everything from depression to cancer. Nurses perform treatments such as reiki, therapeutic touch ("nontherapeutic hovering" as skeptics would define it), massage therapy, and numerous other energy-based techniques. For the most part, though, healing is understood as being controlled by the mind, with an increasing move away from physical care and scientific medicine. For all the postmodern talk about "caring," the health care culture is developing an increasingly impersonal and economically driven health care system. Furthermore, this understanding of health may even allow physician-assisted suicide or euthanasia to become acceptable "therapeutic" means, as experiences in the Netherlands and Oregon testify.

The postmodern worldview lends itself to qualitative research. Both phenomenological and ethnographic research methods are growing in popularity among nurse researchers. If nurse researchers want to know how to define nursing, observe what nurses are doing. If they want to determine the health needs of a population, ask them what they want. To define spirituality, conduct a concept analysis in the nursing literature. This worldview assumes no presuppositions and no absolutes. Conclusions are drawn from conventional wisdom. Qualitative research can be quite useful in identifying trends and even spiritual concerns of those in our care; however, when used to establish truth, difficulties emerge.

A Biblically Informed Worldview

Into this clash of worldviews, parish nurses bring a biblically informed worldview, a Christian theological perspective. Many of us have grown up in the middle of a paradigm shift. To a great extent, we are modernists, heavily swayed by "what the research says." We love it when the research proves that prayer works and that going to church is good for our health. We love the benefits of technology.

On the other hand, we are also postmodernists. We pride ourselves on our tolerance. We hesitate to make value judgments. We do not talk about sin very much anymore. We prefer to think that everyone is basically good—although that becomes more difficult every day as we hear about endless wars and children entering schools with guns. Most of us have tried nutritional supplements of some sort and a host of other unproven therapies "just in case they might work." If something makes us feel better, we assume it must work. Furthermore, we assume that if it makes us feel good, then it must be a gift from God that we should graciously accept and enjoy. However, as Christians in this world of shifting paradigms, we are really a third culture, and we cannot check our theological discernment and critical thinking at the spiritual borders we cross. We worship the Sovereign Lord of the universe. The prophet Isaiah writes:

> For thus says the high and lofty one who inhabits eternity, whose name is Holy: I dwell in the high and holy place, and also with those who are contrite and humble in spirit, to revive the spirit of the humble, and to revive the heart of the contrite. (Isaiah 57:15, NRSV)

This holy God is both immanent and transcendent. No disengaged clockmaker, he created us in his own image to enter into a personal relationship with us—God loves us deeply, intimately, and passionately. This loving creator made us each unique individuals, with wills, intentions, and a propensity to turn away from God to run our own lives. The image of God makes us thinking, feeling, creative persons, but we are not gods or goddesses, and never will be. We cannot presume to be one with God, but instead, defer to him in humble worship and obedience. God has communicated with us through the law, the prophets, and ultimately through his son, Jesus. We have his word preserved for us in the scriptures and illuminated by his spirit, who constantly guides and comforts us.

Furthermore, God has given us the church as his living body. Through the church we find a community that provides love, support, guidance, and a corporate witness to God's love. Through the church his word is preserved, proclaimed, and demonstrated. We are a worshiping community, with our focus on God, who gives perspective to our daily crises and triumphs. We are constantly renewed through word, sacrament, and the "mutual consolation of the saints." We are also a praying community—helping one another stay in close communication with God and our community.

Truth in the biblical worldview is both objective and subjective. Christians can respect and use good science. In fact, it was the Christian faith that desacralized the natural world so that it could be studied. In Christ, we need not fear the spirits of the trees, streams, and ancestors that pagans believed would take vengeance upon them if disturbed. However, truth is not limited to what we can measure or study in a test tube. The biblical worldview takes into account the spiritual realm and the fallen condition of humanity. We learn the truth about human nature and the nature and meaning of the universe from the scriptures. Ultimately, Truth was embodied in the person of Jesus Christ. While Christian faith allows for various interpretations of truth, we acknowledge that, ultimately, Truth is absolute and it rests in God.

The Bible provides insight into our environment that no amount of human reason or observation can discover. First, we learn that it is a created universe, and that God designed it with purpose and meaning. God declared all that he created good, but we also learn that it is polluted by sin. St. Paul writes:

> The creation waits with eager longing for the revealing of the children of God; for the creation was subjected to futility, not of its own will but by the will of the one who subjected it, in hope that the creation itself will be set free from its bondage to decay and will obtain the freedom of the glory of the children of God. (Romans 8:19-21, NRSV)

The physical world is real—not an illusion, as other worldviews may assume. The creation is not God, nor does it contain God. We are not to worship the earth or the stars or the sun. We worship the creator, not the creation. God gave us stewardship over this world, expecting us to be responsible caretakers, and to enjoy the fruits of our labors. However, the problem of sin often makes our work difficult and the results of our efforts uncertain.

The Bible also reveals that an unseen, spiritual realm—which is not neutral—surrounds us. It is inhabited by personal spiritual beings. God is the creator and supreme ruler of this realm, but Satan and his legions have rebelled against God and wage war against him. God forbids humans to attempt contact with the spirit world, except through him, because these spiritual entities are deceitful and seek to manipulate us away from God.

The person in the biblical worldview, beyond being created good in God's image and fallen through sin, is seen as integrated and relational. There is no division between body and soul, but we are embodied spirits, created to live in relationship with God and others. To be healthy means to live as God created us to be. Health itself is found in the concept of *shalom,* a God-centered wholeness that incorporates the ideas of physical, spiritual, and psychosocial well-being, welfare, peace, justice, righteousness, friendship, community, and happiness. Nursing, therefore, becomes compassionate care for the whole person to foster *shalom.* It includes comfort for the dying and active concern for the oppressed and disenfranchised. It is a direct response of overflowing gratitude for God's love.

Nursing research in this worldview becomes a freedom to explore and understand the world God has given us. It can be both qualitative and quantitative, but it is grounded in the presupposition that God not only exists but is present and active in the world today. We look to him for meaning in our research findings. For instance, we can study perceptions of spiritual needs by interviewing nurses or patients, but we must turn to scripture to validate those perceptions. We may show that therapeutic touch raises hemoglobin levels, but we also need to examine its spiritual presuppositions before using it as a healing modality.

Biblically Informed Parish Nursing

Finally, we must ask, what is the nature of the care that parish nurses should provide? Each worldview answers these questions differently. Modernism pushes us to become "professional" and financially savvy. We strive for acceptance and recognition from professional nursing bodies. We expect a salary comparable to colleagues in secular settings. We adopt a taxonomy and an approach set by the marketplace. We seek to protect ourselves legally. On the other hand, postmodernism urges us toward the softer, gentler side of nursing. It exalts spirituality and presence. It tells us to look at the whole person, to be creative in our care. What is more, it give us something concrete we can "do" to meet the needs of those in our care in the form of alternative therapies.

Although we can learn from both the modern and postmodern worldviews, each of them only sees "in part." Neither allows for the fallenness of humanity and creation—which incidentally are comforting doctrines. Our sinful human nature throughout history has corrupted health care into a quest for power and economic gain—regardless of the worldview followed. We need an objective basis for Truth, found in the revelation of God in the Bible, to fully inform our understanding and to give us discernment. Furthermore, we need the power of the Holy Spirit to guide and strengthen us to care for the marginal people of society, to love the unlovely, and to keep going in the face of discouragement.

Jesus illustrated what it means to truly care for our neighbor in the story of the Good Samaritan (Luke 10:30-37). He describes how the Samaritan willingly crossed racial and ethnic barriers, risking his own life, time, and resources to care for a wounded man. While preaching the kingdom of God was Jesus' main mission on earth, he demonstrated his message through physical healing, touch, and human caring. The body was extremely important to Jesus, and, hence, so was physical care.

When we look at parish nursing as an expression of the gospel message, each of these theological concepts shapes the way we practice nursing. We must consider the practical implications of how we view the character of God, the church, the person, the environment, health, and nursing, for our perspectives will determine what kind of parish nurses we will be. Will we continue to offer only "hands off" care, or should we also care for the body? Will we press on for certification and secular recognition, or will we listen more carefully to the church and the scriptures than we do to the call for professional status? Will we reach out to the poor, the disenfranchised, and the culturally diverse, or will we continue to minister primarily to those of our own race, culture, and socioeconomic status?

If we are to be faithful, we will seek to be led by God, rather than by the nursing profession or the culture at large. That might plunge us into conflict, but it might also revolutionize nursing for the better.

REFERENCES

Aikens, C.A. (1924). *Studies in ethics for nurses.* Philadelphia, PA: W.B. Saunders Company.

Barnett, J. M. (1995). *The diaconate: A full and equal order.* Valley Forge, PA: Trinity Press International.

Bullough, B. and Bullough, V.L. (1987). Our roots: What we should know about nursing's Christian pioneers. *Journal of Christian Nursing 4*(1): 11-12.

Burow, D.R. (1985). *Discipleship.* Minneapolis, MN: Augsburg Fortress.

Calabria, M.D. and Macrae, J.A. (1994). *Suggestions for thought by Florence Nightingale.* Philadelphia, PA: University of Pennsylvania Press.

Carson, V.B. (1989). *Spiritual dimensions of nursing practice.* Philadelphia, PA: W.B. Saunders.

Clark, E. (1983). *Women in the early church.* Collegeville, MN: Liturgical Press.

Coakley, M.L. (1989). Florence Nightingale: A one-woman revolution. *Journal of Christian Nursing 6*(1): 20-25.

Descartes, R. (1641/1969). Meditations on first philosophy. In Wolff, R.P., ed., *Ten great works of philosophy* (p. 165). New York: Mentor/Penguin.

Dickens, C. (1868). *Martin Chuzzlewit.* New York and Boston: Books, Inc.

Dock, L.L. and Stewart, I.M. (1931). *A short history of nursing: From the earliest times to the present day.* New York, London: G.P. Putman's Sons, Knickerbocker Press.

Dolan, J., Fitzpatrick, M.L., and Herrmann, E.K. (1983). *Nursing in society: A historical perspective* (Fifteenth edition). Philadelphia, PA: W. B. Saunders.

Donahue, M.P. (1996). *Nursing: The finest art: An illustrated history.* St. Louis, MO: C.V. Mosby.

Gleick, J. (1999). Untitled. *Time, 153*(12): 78.

Haazig, M. (1989). Historical presence of the nurse in the church. *Oneness in purpose—diversity in practice: Third annual Granger Westberg parish nurse symposium.* Park Ridge, IL: National Parish Nurse Resource Center.

Hamilton, D. (1994). Constructing the mind of nursing. *Nursing History Review, 2:* 3-28.

Hensley, D., Kilgore, K.A., Langfitt, J.V., and Peterson, L. (1986). Margaret Newman model of health. In Ann Marriner, ed., *Nursing theorists and their work* (p. 371). St. Louis, MO: Mosby.

McNeill, R.H. (1910). The ideal nurse. *American Journal of Nursing 10*(3): 393.

Parse, R.R. (1995). *Illuminations: The human becoming theory in practice and research.* New York: National League for Nursing Press.

Rogers, M.E. (1983). The science of unitary human beings: A paradigm for nursing. In Clements, I.W. and Roberts, F.B. *Family Health: A Theoretical Approach to Nursing Care.* New York: John Wiley.

Watson, J. (1994). A frog, a rock, a ritual: Myth, mystery, and metaphors for an ecocaring cosmology in a universe that is turning over. In Schuster, E.A. and Brown, C.L. (eds.), New York: National League for Nursing Press, 17-39.

Wentz, A.R. (1936). *Fliedner the faithful.* Philadelphia, PA: The Board of Publication of the United Lutheran Church in America.

Widerquist, J. (1992). Florence Nightingale's calling. *Second Opinion 17*(3): 108-121.

Widerquist, J. (1995). Called to serve. *Christian Nurse International 11*(1): 5.

Zersen, D. (1994). Parish nursing: 20th century fad? *Journal of Christian Nursing 11*(2).

SECTION III:
PREPARATION FOR PARISH NURSING—
SPIRITUAL FORMATION AND CLINICAL
PASTORAL EDUCATION

Chapter 4

Spiritual Formation for Parish Nursing

Sandra Thomas

Parish nursing, as all forms of ministry, does not consist of techniques and programs; it is a compassionate heart and an educated mind working together to meet the challenge of the moment.

Sandra Thomas

INTRODUCTION

We had been warned. "An educational program for parish nurses will attract a large number of students and their personal issues will dominate the process." The design team was in the middle of a year-long effort to develop a curriculum for the preparation of parish nurses. Although we appreciated the warning, it did not come as new information. It was true; we could anticipate students enrolling in a parish nursing course for many reasons other than a pure intention to serve God and humanity. Students enroll because they are experiencing burnout as nurses, because they want to find a way to "witness" to patients, because they are frustrated and angry with changes in the health care system, or because they are fascinated with alternative medicine. Some bring a subconscious desire to occupy a position of influence in their congregation. Many come seeking some resolution to their personal spiritual struggles.

The design team was also aware that persons not suited to the ministry of parish nursing would apply. No doubt, we would turn most of our applicants away if we accepted only those who were spiritually and emotionally mature, who were free of personal neediness or unresolved questioning. None of us knew any such nurses. In fact, we did not know any faculty members, clergy, chaplains, doctors, social workers, or pastoral counselors who functioned with such maturity.

The reality is, people are drawn to caring vocations out of their own pain and struggle. Thus, rather than heed the warning about needy students, we chose to recognize their wounds as potential strengths that could, in most cases, be reframed and healed through spiritual formation. The witness of scripture reveals God's willingness to work through less than perfect individuals. Over and over those stories reveal not only that God works through "unfinished" people but that those persons grow and are changed in the process.

Our reflection on how God "selects" ministry candidates (e.g., parish nursing students) led to an important addition in our curriculum design. Students enrolled not only in a course but also in a spiritual formation experience that focused on call and vocation, exploring the journeys of others whom God had recruited and trained. They then reflected on their own sense of call, both in class and in written assignments. The warnings we had received about wounded students led the design team to add a fifth dimension to the four traditional dimensions of "call."[1] Echoing the writings of Henri Nouwen (1979), we would teach students and remind ourselves that God's call to us often comes at the point of our own woundedness.

Clergy and chaplains know that the call to ministry comes in part from spiritual emptiness or grows out of a desire to provide for others the care we long for ourselves. In the same way, nurses are often (although not always) drawn to their profession by early experiences of helplessness in the face of tragedy, including the illness or death of a significant person. To some extent that helpless feeling is addressed through our education. Knowing what to do, when, where, and how builds confidence and a valuable competence.

Many nurses embrace their "call to nursing" as a divinely appointed vocation. For them, nursing is a ministry, an exciting opportunity not only to help others but also to build relationships and empower individuals and families. For these nurses, caring is process and technique rather than technique alone.

Often such nurses enroll in our parish nursing courses. They come feeling called to something more as nurses. They come with pain inflicted by the frustrations of a changing health care system that limits them to the use of techniques and excludes relationships. They have seen people who needed more care, who need the care they want very much to provide. The most frustrating difficulty is that nurses interact with patients through specific helping acts (e.g., blood pressure screening) and not in long-term relationships.

Nothing engenders more feelings of helplessness than a long-term caring relationship with a person perceived as body, mind, and spirit. It is quite different to tell people they have high blood pressure than it is to journey with them as they fail in attempts to change their lifestyle, as family members and church potluck dinners undo their frail resolve, and as the questions change from the "how" of biology to the "why" of theology.

That feeling of helplessness challenges the best of us. Parish nursing students who do not have their own lives in order, who have deep spiritual questions, who fail in their own attempts to live healthy lives are not students we should turn away. Their pain is not a handicap to learning, but rather a wonderful teachable moment! It creates openness to spiritual formation where our failure, sin, and helpless feelings are engaged and transformed.

In this chapter we examine what spiritual formation seeks to accomplish and how this experience can be incorporated into the basic preparation for parish nursing. Nursing education contains parallel experiences that constitute bridges for persons adding ministry to their profession of nursing. We describe those bridges. Finally, we examine how clergy, chaplains, and parish nurses can mutually support one another in a lifelong process of spiritual formation.

Those of us who work with suffering persons need more than a few good techniques. We need to be prepared for and continually engaged in a spiritual formation process that helps us find within our own relationship to God and the church a "balm in Gilead."[2]

SPIRITUAL FORMATION

Roman Catholic seminary education has long used the concept of spiritual formation, and it is now becoming more familiar to Protestants. Its process guides students on an inner journey intended to identify and develop their gifts for ministry. Along with academic instruction, formation molds and shapes students, and future parish nurses, into informed professionals with hearts for ministry that trust the guidance of the Holy Spirit. It lays the foundation for ongoing growth that values the process and seeks out supportive relationships, welcomes mentors, and practices spiritual disciplines. The process of spiritual formation led a student to say at the end of a parish nurse preparation program, "This course was a life changing experience for me."

In 1996, the Association of Theological Schools affirmed the importance of spiritual formation in preparation for ministry through further development of accrediting standards. Those standards now state that, in preparing men and women for ministry, theological schools must "provide opportunities for formational experiences through which students may grow in those personal qualities essential for the practice of ministry, namely, emotional maturity, personal faith, moral integrity, and social concern." These are the same personal qualities needed by parish nurses who serve congregations—emotional maturity, personal faith, moral integrity, and social concern.

The Scope of Spiritual Formation—Personal Formation

To examine how chaplains, congregational clergy, and parish nurses can support one another in ongoing spiritual formation, it is helpful to define the dimensions of the process. Daniel O. Aleshire (1999), Executive Director to the Association of Theological Schools, in an interview with *Christian Century* magazine, outlines three dimensions in spiritual formation. The first is personal formation. One needs maturity and interpersonal skills to function successfully in a job that is primarily relational. This has long been recognized in nursing, and the processes used to form professional identity in nursing parallel the process of personal formation for ministry.

Developing a professional identity as "minister" is one of the most important and difficult transitions from traditional nursing to parish nursing. Being present as a pastor is much different from caring for the patient in a surgical recovery room. After studying the *Scope and Standards of Parish Nursing Practice* (Health Ministries Association and American Nurses Association, 1998), it is not uncommon to hear a student ask in a plaintive voice, "If a person needs a dressing changed and I'm not supposed do it, what am I supposed to do?" It is a question that supervisors in clinical pastoral education (CPE) encounter frequently. The formation processes developed in the training of chaplains are valuable components of education for parish nursing.[3]

Other aspects of personal formation and professional identity are familiar to nurses. Nursing educators have long known that mastery of facts and procedures alone does not make a good nurse any more than mastery of Greek and Hebrew makes a good pastor. The personal character a nurse brings to each encounter and the inner abilities required to care and to cope are equally essential.

Relationship skill and professional identity are more important in parish nursing than in most other types of nursing because it is an independent practice. Parish nurses must have the professional maturity to structure their practice, set priorities, establish boundaries, initiate contacts, and make decisions without an immediate supervisor. A freedom and a burden of responsibility exist that are common to clergy, chaplains, and parish nurses. The freedom is to structure one's time and decide the depth of one's involvement in any particular situation. The responsibility is the power of our presence, words, and acts in the lives of those we serve.

Moving from a "dependent practice" in which one follows directives set by others to an "independent practice" in which one decides which priorities will establish the day's work is one of the most stressful transitions in nursing (Murray, 1998). Even in uncomplicated encounters with patients, nurses experience high levels of stress and recidivism when making home visits that require their independent judgment and decision making. Parish nursing is an independent practice, and developing a level of comfort and confidence in working independently is an essential element of professional development.

Journal writing is an important part of a nursing student's first clinical experience because it builds on the power of personal encounter (Kobert, 1995). It encourages students to give explicit attention to their own emotions and to observe how their actions impact patients. Journals provide a safe place for describing worries, fears, doubt, and feelings of inadequacy that are a normal part of learning a profession. In addition, writing offers students an opportunity to reflect on alternate ways of responding. Faculty members reading and responding to journal entries have opportunities to invite the exploration of issues and concerns unique to the individual student.

As a familiar practice, journal writing is easily incorporated into education for parish nursing. As a course requirement, journaling conveys the importance of reflecting on experience, allowing a safe avenue for expressing emotion. When journal writings are shared with a faculty member over two semesters and elicit written responses from the faculty, the journal develops into a personalized "mentoring" conversation that encourages growth in personal maturity for the student.

Small-group reflection is a personal formation experience common to both nursing education (Davies, 1995) and the education of chaplains. Chaplains bring valuable skills to an ongoing reflection group for parish nurses. Parish nurses bring valuable insights for chaplains! Many nurses have experienced small-group reflective learning as part of their first clinical experience in a faculty-led peer group (Carkhuff, 1996).

The challenge for chaplains or clergy who lead reflection groups with parish nurses is that nursing consultation groups tend to be solution oriented. Turning attention away from problem solving will require serious effort on the part of chaplains or theological faculty members. Peter Buttitta (1995) has developed a case consultation process for parish nurses that can be very useful. Participation in case consultation demands some degree of personal maturity. That maturity deepens as parish nurses discover the value of their presence, realize how they are changed by encounters with parishioners, and reflect on the ways God may be acting in and through this situation.

Small-group reflection becomes a resource and experience that many parish nurses continue beyond their basic training because it helps them make the transition from hospital or office settings into independent parish nurse practices. Moving into parish nursing is similar to beginning home care nursing, a transition known to be very stressful with a high rate of recidivism. Recognizing the difficulty, parish clergy and chaplains can offer support. They, in turn, will benefit from seeing their ministry setting through fresh eyes.

Other experiences that contribute to personal formation include building relationships with faculty, clergy, and chaplains who model the type of pastoral behavior necessary in parish nurses—a healthy attitude toward parishioners, congregational life, and the work of ministry. They must model healthy relationship skills, demonstrate an ability to manage conflict, and willingly share their own faith or spiritual struggles. For some parish nurses, finding such a mentor will be their first personal encounter with a mature religious leader.

The Scope of Spiritual Formation—Learning the Culture

The second ingredient in spiritual formation is learning the culture and traditions of a religious denomination (Aleshire, 1999). Many parish nurses have negotiated their way through the culture of the hospital world and will need to do so again in the congregation, their new practice environment. Congregations have their own culture, traditions, power structure, and symbolic acts. Parish nurses need to understand how to "work the system," what boundaries exist in the religious community, and what policies and traditions apply to them. Parish nurses may discover that the same territorial struggles they previously experienced at the hospital or clinic also take place in their church. Checking blood pressures after worship services will require permission. Nurses who have baptized babies in the hospital nursery when the infant was in danger of dying need to investigate how their own Lutheran, Baptist, Presbyterian, or Roman Catholic church would respond to the parish nurse baptizing an infant. Parish nurses who visit new parents must be prepared for questions about how, in their particular congregation, one prepares for baptism, dedication, and worshiping with an infant.

Parish nurses need the opportunity to learn how the congregation they serve expresses its faith theologically. They will want to respond genuinely to spiritual concerns, using words that are meaningful in that particular tradition, dealing maturely with their own doubts, questions, and spiritual "folklore" in order to respond to the needs of the people they serve.

Most denominations offer a world of resources that are new to nurses. Our students are surprised to learn that their denominations have taken social stands on end-of-life care, have videotaped programs on caring for the elderly, or have a national office that relates to parish nursing. Students must learn what is distinctive about their own denominational beliefs and rituals, what is appropriate work for a parish nurse, the resources of the denomination and what is available in terms of prayer and ritual, and the work style of the clergy on the staff of their congregation. A nurse's own pastor, priest, or rabbi can be extremely helpful in this area.

Chaplains can make important contributions to parish nurses also. They have learned how to care for a diverse population with ethnic, social, and cultural differences. They have valuable experiences and resources to share with parish nurses concerning people from various faith traditions or from no faith tradition at all. Learning the culture and traditions of the various faiths and denominations gives one confidence, resources, and authority in presence.

One other difficult transition merits discussion. Meeting the congregation as a "human institution" often brings disappointment and a deep sense of loss. Parish nurses discover that "behind the scenes" clergy can be difficult, uncaring, and self-absorbed; the church secretary can be irritable, the musician can be territorial, and the whole congregation can display little interest in becoming "healthy God-fearing people." This represents the loss of the idealistic image of church as a holy place, as well as the loss of the perfect parental figure to whom one can turn for unconditional love and support. Clergy and chaplains have experienced this transition themselves and can help interpret it for parish nurses to support them in their grieving process.

The Scope of Spiritual Formation—Personal Faith

Finally, the dimension identified by Aleshire (1999) that comes first to mind when we say "spiritual formation" is developing a well-defined, personal, active faith. Formal nursing education possesses no parallel to this. Hopefully, however, students come to a parish nurse education course with the expectation that they will learn how to share faith with others.

Theological schools have learned that students bring with them a faith culture that they can articulate but that is not very functional. Part of the theological education process is gently taking a student's heritage apart and putting it back together in a way that informs the heart. Parish nurses do not have the benefit of three or four years of theological education, but they must undertake the same faith transformation.

Some nurses have done this inner spiritual work already in the face of their experiences with suffering people. They have wrestled with the questions that have no answers, they have turned to prayer as a personal resource, and they have questioned and refined their inherited faith tradition into a meaningful personal spiritual center. Not unlike ministry students, other nurses come with a yet-to-be-tested "Sunday school" faith. Attention given to faith development and autobiographical reflection helps one begin to see life as sacred text. Parish nurses who would lead others on a spiritual journey must discover how they themselves have been wounded and blessed, how they have been twisted and strengthened by their own spiritual journey.

An experience of "community" is vital for parish nurses because they serve in the most intricate and dynamic of all communities. Essential to their ministry is the ability to "be there" for one another, to understand God as active in the midst of the community, and to experience the community as caregiver. Parish nurses minister not only to individuals but also to the congregation as a whole. The power of life in the dynamic system called "congregation" requires more than book learning; it requires learning from personally receiving the care of others in the church, from the awe and a deep appreciation formed by one's experience in community.

CONCLUSION

In nursing, as in ministry, we have passed through a time of renewed interest in what it means to be "professional." Much attention is given to producing informed and skilled professionals. The amount of information required to practice in a dual profession such as parish nursing is overwhelming. It demands a constant intake of information. Even as we master the facts, we need also to attend to the type of inner character developing in those who serve us at times of utmost vulnerability. To take on nursing as a ministry requires spiritual formation that wrestles with the deep issues of life and emerges as an ability to attend to others and speak about faith. It is a spirit both formed and informed by colleagues, patients, parishioners, fine mentors, and quality instruction. It is a spirit both formed in the humility that comes from living in a community rich in faith tradition and wealthy in human sharing.

NOTES

1. Historically the church has defined *call* as a convergence of (a) our inner sense of God's call to us, (b) demonstrated gifts and graces for the work to which we are being called, (c) the affirmation of our call by the congregation or denomination, and (d) an opportunity to serve.

2. The phrase "a balm in Gilead," made popular by the American folk hymn, comes from Jeremiah 8:22. The prophet Jeremiah is mourning for his people, lost in pain and despair that encompasses body, mind, soul, relationships, and communal safety. The hymn responds, "There is a balm in Gilead to make the wounded whole. . . ."

3. While structured differently than clinical pastoral education groups, the training for chaplains invites students to explore (a) feelings and ideas, (b) reflect on their practice of new skills, (c) receive clarification and validation, (d) learning the processes of working in a team, and (e) refocus on the needs of the client.

REFERENCES

Aleshire, D. (1999). Seminaries and the ecology of faith: An interview with Daniel Aleshire. *Christian Century,* February 3-10, 110-123.

The Association of Theological Schools (1996). *Accreditation standards.* Available online at <www.ats.edu>.

Buttitta, P. (1985). Theological reflection in health ministry: A strategy for parish nurses. In J. Whitehead and E. Whitehead (eds.), *Theological Reflection and Christian Ministry* (pp. 112-122). New York: Harper SanFrancisco.

Carkhuff, M. (1996). Reflective learning: Work groups as learning groups. *The Journal of Continuing Education in Nursing, 5,* 209-214.

Davies, E. (1995). Reflective practice: A focus for caring. *Journal of Nursing Education, 34*(4), 167-174.

Health Ministries Association and American Nurses Association (1998). *Scope and standards of parish nursing practice.* Washington, DC: American Nurses Publishing.

Kobert, L. (1995). In our own voice: Journaling as a teaching/learning technique for nurses. *Journal of Nursing Education, 34*(3), 140-142.

Murray, T. (1998). Using role theory concepts to understand transitions from hospital-based nursing practice to home care nursing. *The Journal of Continuing Education in Nursing, 29*(3), 105-111.

Nouwen, Henri J.M. (1979). *The wounded healer.* New York: Doubleday and Company, Inc.

Chapter 5

A Mystical Understanding
of Clinical Pastoral Education

Larry Austin

And there came a leper to him, beseeching him, and kneeling down to
him, and saying to him,
    If you will,
        you can make me clean.
And Jesus moved with compassion,
    put forth his hand,
    touched him,
    and said to him, I will;
Be thou clean.

(Mark 1:40-41)

This chapter presents an understanding of clinical pastoral education (CPE), an experiential theological education process. CPE grew
out of the intensive discussions early in the twentieth century that examined the value and efficacy of America's medical and theological
educational institutions (Thornton, 1970). In the field of medical education, the Flexner Report (1910) led to legislative acts that improved
the quality of medical education. At the same time, a variety of religious authorities were reforming seminary education as well. Thornton (1970) quotes William Palmer Ladd in an address to the General
Convention of the Protestant Episcopal Church in 1913 as follows:

> The theological courses in our seminaries need to be supple-
> mented by some kind of practical training. We all know how we
> found ourselves the week after our graduation and ordination

face to face with problems with which our seminary course had not prepared us to deal. Most of us floundered across the gulf and sooner or later got on our feet, but with some of us it was later rather than sooner, and only after costly and perhaps bitter experience. Can we not do something to eliminate this waste? (p. 31)

Several groups of pastoral educators struggled for years to increase the viability of seminary education. Some wanted to hold theological education to the same scientific rigor being applied to medical education; others resisted such efforts. Several Protestant groups established training programs for seminary students that provided diverse, unique, and practical training. The most influential programs contained hands-on training in ministry to persons in need, coupled with the student's focused reflection on ministry.

These ministry training programs carried on their activities side by side and had little interaction until the late 1940s when representatives began to meet. After twenty years of consultation, the Council of Clinical Training, the Institute of Pastoral Care, the Southern Baptist Association for Clinical Pastoral Education, and the Lutheran Advisory Council on Pastoral Care merged in 1967 into the Association of Clinical Pastoral Education, Inc. This new association became the standard-setting, accrediting, and certifying body for the clinical theological education of students.

It would be easy to focus this chapter on the history or logical components of CPE. Program requirements, objectives, and outcomes of introductory or supervisory education are available from the central office of the association.[1] However, this historical and logical approach would not capture the profound sense of wonderment that many have experienced.

Theology may be described as an articulation of the content of religious faith in a coherent and logical form. Pastoral theology concerns itself with the practical discipline of ministry. The rational or logical understanding of God or the holy has always seemed somewhat inadequate to me. Faith and its expression so often seem more irrational and illogical, particularly in institutional ministry with its ongoing chaos. Thus, to speak of faith's rational theological understanding does not adequately capture the sense of awe so often experienced in the CPE process. For many students, CPE is a mystical experience, mysticism being defined here as "the belief that direct knowledge of God, spiritual truth, or ultimate reality can be attained through subjective experience" (*Webster's Ninth New Collegiate Dictionary,* 1984). For some of us, such experiences have permanently impacted our life's journey in ministry. This journey began in our early lives and was enhanced with CPE. Historically, we reflect upon our religious faith by the interactions of tradition, holy readings, and narratives. These methods help us understand who we are, where we came from, and what we are to become. As we share the narratives of our faith, we all participate in the life journey of others. This mutual sharing builds community and helps us develop our own sense of tradition and reflections of faith. These reflections are passed on through our personal interpretations and that helps the next generation develop its understandings, traditions, and narratives.

Mystics often tell us that people teach us about life. CPE has its own set of narratives and traditions about life's journeys. CPE places us in actual ministry situations where we encounter people and the holy. In a more personal way, CPE helped me reflect upon my story and how my story parallels others that I have encountered. It is my contention that the mystical theology inherent in people's stories makes CPE what it is. As we understand our stories, we become sensitized to the lives of others around us.

Learning about the complexities of our lives, we also learn about the complexities of others'. In CPE I have encountered some stories so fantastic that they are almost unbelievable. Some of the stories are no doubt metaphorical, or apocryphal; some may even be literal and true. My point is, all the stories I have encountered have worth and value. Active reflection about people, their traditions, and their stories has taught me much in my learning process.

I began my CPE journey in 1974, and in subsequent years realized a single and powerful truth about every student and supervisor whom I have encountered: we all love to tell stories about our experiences. When a group of students and supervisors gather, we quickly digress into stories about our experiences in supervision, patient ministry, certification committees, and other aspects of our institutional lives. The memories are powerful and sometimes traumatic. Some of our stories are funny, some painful, some frustrating, but rarely are they forgettable. With that introduction, let me tell you a story.

My first CPE unit was in a psychiatric hospital. On my first day, I dutifully appeared on my assigned unit of severely disturbed adults and somehow made my way into the dayroom. As I observed the patients moving about, I felt very alone. An older man suddenly appeared by my side and asked, "Are you the new chaplain?" I replied, "Am I that obvious?" He went on to talk to me a while about the fact that he had been in the institution for a considerable time and had learned to recognize new people, especially chaplains. As we talked I noticed my anxiety decreased somewhat, even though I still could not tell if the old man was a staff member or patient. After a short while he leaned toward me, pointed his finger at the patients in the dayroom, and, in a conspiratorial tone asked, "Chaplain, do you know the difference between you and me and those patients over there?" Having no response but my silence, he withdrew a set of keys from his pocket, jangled them in front of my face, and uttered one word: "Keys." As he turned and resumed mopping the floor, I realized that my supervisor had given us an orientation but no keys. Supervision of my ministry had begun before I ever had my first group or individual supervision session. Students reflect about their work in unlikely places and learn unexpected lessons from people who, we naively assume, have nothing to offer.

The CPE stories I have heard usually contain four main reference points:

- An element of surprise
- A sense of awareness
- Anxiety-producing vulnerability
- Graceful insight

Religious faith systems have their own stories as well and often have the same points of reference. Denominations, faith traditions, and religious groups pass on their teachings and traditions through oral stories and written scriptures. In my faith tradition, the cleansing of the leper is an important story. This narrative, quoted at the beginning of this chapter, captures for me some of the practical issues that we find in modern health care. This story's dynamics also closely parallel some CPE learning experiences.

Lepers were considered unclean and thus excluded from family, community, and worship in the temple. We constantly encounter people in our institutions who are estranged from their communities. Their pain often drives them to extreme behaviors, and they seek to be heard and understood in their darkest moments. The underlying pastoral issue in the story of the leper is one of restoration or reconciliation back into the community of family, faith, and society. In pastoral care, much of our work deals with reconciliation of these same issues.

This leper was crafty. He somehow got close enough to Jesus to confront him face-to-face. It must have been quite a surprise for the crowd to realize that they were in the presence of one who was "unclean."

The CPE process constantly surprises the beginning student. Students voice their surprise by talking about the overwhelming amount of paperwork required, or the picky supervisor, or how unrealistic it is to remember all those interchanges for the verbatim. The biggest surprise is often from the patients themselves and the feelings that these encounters stir up within us. One never knows exactly what to expect when working with human beings in the chaos and crisis of the moment. The learning intensifies greatly when the student, expecting to deal with only the patient dynamic, is surprised to learn that his or her own chaos may be the true learning issue. Ekstein and Wallerstein (1972) describe this as the difference between "learning problems" (student-client relationships) and "problems about learning" (student-supervisor relationships).

A new student assigned to an orthopedic unit visited patients for about an hour and then angrily entered the supervisor's office. She exclaimed, "How did you know that I hate to work with alcoholics? The first three patients I saw confessed to me that they were alcoholics, and you know how many issues I have with people like that." Surprise happened for both the student and the supervisor.

The student expected to find orthopedic patients on the orthopedic unit, not people with alcohol problems. The student was surprised at the intensity of her feelings; she thought she had them under better control. She also was surprised (angry/fearful/threatened) at her perception of the supervisor's uncanny ability to see her issues so clearly and quickly. The student was definitely disconcerted and scared. It was unnerving to think herself so transparent that the supervisor had set learning in motion even before she saw her first patient.

The supervisor was equally surprised. He did not remember reading anything in the student's materials that identified specific problems with any particular type of patient or issue. He was somewhat surprised by the student's perception of his great power. The supervisor was tempted for a moment to let the student believe that he really was that insightful. However, he chose to talk to the student about coincidence and/or providence of the placement. As supervision progressed throughout the unit, the student and supervisor both had to deal with their preconceived conceptions of reality. They had to grapple with their idealized perceptions of the patients, the nature of the institution, and their supervisory relationship (Horney, 1945).

The leper asked for cleansing, not healing. He conceded the fact that Jesus had the power to cleanse. The leper's confrontation was about willingness, not power. Jesus heard accurately, was motivated by compassion, and was vulnerable. He responded congruently to the leper's request by willingly addressing his issue. He touched the leper and he said, "I will; Be thou clean." Jesus was aware and vulnerable. In his touching of the leper, Jesus became one with the unclean. We do not have any record of emotional reactions of anyone at this point in this story, but I am willing to opine that emotions were intense to say the least.

Following the admission of their first AIDS patient, who was in fact a hospital employee, considerable discussion took place at various administrative levels, exploring the proper response to this person. In one discussion, a high-ranking administrator suggested that it would not look good for this religiously based hospital to admit a staff member with AIDS. He thought that it might be better to send the patient to another hospital. The chaplain involved in the meeting was aghast at this attitude and spoke passionately against the transfer. Following the chaplain's recommendation, the group decided that the patient would stay. After the meeting, the infection control nurse asked the chaplain to visit the patient because she felt the chaplain's visit would be helpful. The chaplain felt affirmed by her own stand against injustice and by the confidence of the nurse. While putting on the infection control gown, mask, gloves, booties, and cap, the chaplain wondered what it would be like to pray in a mask. She believed that she had been asked to make this visit and knew that God was somehow giving her an opportunity to perform a significant ministry. After the chaplain had visited and prayed with the patient, she began to move toward the door. The patient said, in a still, small voice, "Chaplain, the next time you come to visit, you don't have to wear the mask." The chaplain instantly became aware of her fear and her conceit, of her similarity to the administrator. As she fled from the room, her awareness filled her with guilt and shame. She wrote up her experience and presented it to her peers in the verbatim group. Her vulnerability and awareness of her own dynamics made the verbatim presentation a painful one. Having responded with good intentions, she was chagrined to learn that she was not as aware as she had envisioned. Through this sharing of her pain, we all experienced the conviction of William James (1958) when he said, over 100 years ago, "The sanest of us are at one with prison inmates and lunatics and death runs the robust of us down" (p. 53). It is a sobering thought to realize that we are not as competent as we might have hoped.

Most of us go through life largely unconscious. We feel, think, respond; we also have a wonderful way of living in denial and keeping many feelings and thoughts at a distance. We are well adapted to a life filled with defenses that keep us safe and protected from our innermost turmoil. Working closely with people in crisis often raises our own unresolved issues.

Having to write verbatims and present them for supervision requires more courage than we ever dreamed, yet that is what CPE requires us to do. In group and individual supervision, students are expected to gain awareness of themselves and their ministry. Supervisors require students to present materials to their peers and receive feedback, whether they want it or not. We interact with students and expect them to risk being vulnerable. Their failures, their pain, and their successes are displayed so that they might learn. This is not an easy task. To bare one's soul to a group of peers and supervisors about one's function in personal ministry and have them provide feedback raises one's anxiety no small degree. When coupled with the anxiety inherent in the patient encounter, the intensity of the CPE experience is easy to see. Real ministry to real people in crisis and realistic reflection on that ministry is not for the fainthearted.

The final point of reference is about graceful insight. CPE students do some really stupid things in training and ministry. I speak from firsthand experience. I took a unit in an intermediate care facility for the retarded. One patient never acknowledged my presence when visited. I grew increasingly challenged and resolved to do something with this patient to get him somehow to respond to me. Commandeering an autoharp from the chaplain's office, I camped out in the patient's room. Having no musical ability did not deter me as I played, sang, and made noise for about an hour. Eventually, I grew tired. As I left, I reached out and touched this resident on the chest and he smiled. I was surprised and immediately sought out my supervisor and told him of my visit. He began to laugh, and the more I told him, the more amused he became. He asked with tears in his eyes if I had read the chart, and when I replied no, he almost fell off his chair. In between his bursts of laughter he told me that the patient was deaf and blind and did not even know I was there until I touched him. I felt like such a fool! It did not help my fragile ego that my respected supervisor was having trouble catching his breath from laughter. After a while, he turned to me and said, "That is the best example of pastoral presence I have ever seen."

The supervisor was able to say that grace-filled thing to me. I was surprised, affirmed, confused, and intrigued. He showed me a way to validate my imperfections with grace. I learned that in my deepest embarrassment, another person was able to find some good in me. This, too, is CPE, and it is my belief that this is what keeps most of us coming back. The painful steps of surprise, awareness, and vulnerability are made bearable by insight enlightened by grace. At times I have felt the confrontation of my peers, supervisors, patients, and their families. It is not easy to admit one's shortcomings, nor to bring them to the group for discussion. It becomes a mystical experience when we realize that there can be no insight, no grace, no understanding, no support, unless we share our vulnerabilities.

CPE is governed by a set of standards that ensure that every program works from the same objectives. Each program has component parts centered on the learning contract, didactics, verbatim studies, interpersonal group, professional readings, and individual supervision. For most CPE students, this is a somewhat familiar exercise. We have for the most part been involved in the pursuit of academic and logical goals most of our lives. The mystical part of CPE challenges us to do more than just think; we are to reflect on feelings as well. The complexities of life are endless and unique. In our search for the holy we find imperfect people in desperate situations. As we enter into relationships with these imperfect people, we somehow find what it was we were seeking.

Specialized ministry has no ways to control what one encounters in the visitation of patients. Just as the leper surprised Jesus, the patients we serve constantly surprise us. We assume that the student will be surprised, and the student is expected to be anxious and vulnerable. Students are expected to share some of their most private thoughts and feelings, reflect on their vulnerabilities, and become aware of their dynamics. It is in this moment of vulnerable reflection that one encounters the holy. We experience a sense of awe about the nature of how God works and learn that awe both inspires and frightens us. If we are lucky to have enlightened supervisors and peers, we find grace and insight as well. CPE can be intimidating, intense, and frightening. It can also be transforming.

I hope that every person who engages in CPE has a positive learning experience. It is different from every other learning experience you will encounter. As a practical and mystical journey into the depths of the human and divine encounter, CPE has the ability to transform lives and will impact your ministry forever. You will certainly come away from the experience with some wonderful stories to tell.

NOTE

1. The Association for Clinical Pastoral Education, Inc., 1549 Clairmont Road, Suite 103, Decatur, GA 30033; phone: (404) 320-1472; fax: (404) 320-0849; e-mail: <acpe@acpe.edu>; Web page: <www.acpe.edu>.

REFERENCES

Ekstein, Rudolf and Wallerstein, Robert (1972). *The teaching and learning of psychotherapy.* New York: International Universities Press, Inc.
Flexner, Abraham (1910). *Medical education in the United States and Canada: A report to the Carnegie Foundation for the Advancement of Teaching.* Bulletin # 4.

Horney, Karen (1945). *Our inner conflicts.* New York: W.W. Norton and Company.

James, William (1958). *The varieties of religious experience.* New York: New American Library.

Thornton, Edward (1970). *Professional education for the ministry.* Nashville, TN: Abingdon Press.

Webster's Ninth New Collegiate Dictionary (1984). Springfield, MA: Merriam-Webster, Inc.

Chapter 6

Parish Nursing and Clinical
Pastoral Education

Paul Derrickson

In 1988, eight parish nurses approached the author's Department of Pastoral Care, expressing an interest in contracting for an introductory unit of clinical pastoral education (CPE). They were concerned that they were losing their spiritual roots.

Their request came at an opportune time. The local health care market was changing from a fee-for-service system to capitation, bringing an increasing percentage of business through managed care contracts. These changes meant that hospitals were looking to the communities for health promotion, illness prevention, and posthospital follow-up care. The role of chaplains as community liaisons took on increasing importance. In that context, the administration granted permission for a parish nurse CPE program that did not require clinical time in the hospital with patients and family members.

DEVELOPING THE PROGRAM

Two planning meetings were held to discuss the requirements of CPE, including the time commitments, the clinical sites, and learning contracts. The author initiated discussions by creating a tentative schedule and providing copies of the Standards of the Association for Clinical Pastoral Education (ACPE) (ACPE, 2000). The parish nurses, in turn, talked about the type of program they sought.

These discussions led to a second meeting in which we agreed on a tentative schedule with the understanding that we would regularly review its content. The schedule stipulated that we meet Friday mornings from 8:00 a.m. to 1:00 p.m. with no meetings on the Fridays following Thanksgiving. With a two-week break during the Christmas holiday, the program ran from September 11, 1998, to April 16, 1999.

Full ACPE applications were required, including admission interviews. The congregations associated with each nurse served as training sites, signed a contract with the CPE program, and (most often) paid the $400 tuition fee. Students reported their clinical hours monthly. A few students anticipated that they would be unable to complete the 300 hours during the scheduled classes and they began their clinical hours during the summer.

THE PROGRAM

Format

The program each Friday consisted of five parts, beginning with opening devotions, brief attention to administrative concerns, and a didactic presentation. A student then presented a verbatim in a very structured format. Students identified the following:

- The facts or content communicated in the visit
- The dynamics or feelings behind the facts and content
- The developmental stages and issues active in the conversation based on Erikson's stages of faith (1963), modified by the feminist critique (Gilligan, 1982)
- Any political, ethical, or social issues
- The theological issues based on Pruyser's (1976) seven diagnostic categories
- A one-sentence pastoral summary

After discussing their one-sentence summary, the student presented a pastoral care plan. The pastoral summary proved the most difficult. Often they tried to combine the diagnosis with a treatment plan. Helping students split the two functions allowed more flexibility in planning various deliberate strategies rather than reflexive responses. After a brief break, the remainder of the time was given to a non-agenda interpersonal group (IPG) experience. Often there were strong links between the didactic, verbatim, and the IPG discussions. The didactic, verbatim, and IPG schedules are described in Table 6.1.

TABLE 6.1. The Proposed CPE Curriculum for Parish Nurses

Week	9:00-10:15 a.m.	10:15-11:15 a.m.	11:30 a.m.-1:00 p.m.
1	Learning Contract	MBTI	IPG
2	Listening Skills	Verbatim	IPG
3	The Sender	Verbatim	IPG
4	The Receiver: Counseling Response	Verbatim	IPG
5	Crisis Intervention Verbatim	IPG	Tacit Contracts
6	Stress, Change, and Self-Care	Verbatim	IPG
7	Systems Theory	Verbatim	IPG
8	Anxiety	Verbatim	IPG
9	Life Cycle	Verbatim	IPG
10	Family Life Cycle	Verbatim	IPG
11	Genogram	Verbatim	IPG
12	Parish Dynamics and Rumors		
13	Midterm Evaluations		
14	Negotiating Role	Verbatim	IPG
15	Spiritual Assessment	Verbatim	IPG
16	Substance Abuse	Verbatim	IPG
17	Suicide	Verbatim	IPG
18	Depression/Loneliness	Verbatim	IPG
19	Aging	Verbatim	IPG
20	Dying, Grief	Verbatim	IPG
21	Spiritual Interventions I	Verbatim	IPG
22	Spiritual Interventions II		
23	Community Resources	Verbatim	IPG
24	Congregational Assessment and Program Development	IPG	
25	Final Evaluations . . . . Graduation		

Note: IPG = interpersonal group; MBTI = Myers-Briggs Type Indicator.

The training program day ended with time for prayer requests, discussion of curricula for the upcoming weeks, and a closing prayer. The first week of the program we each selected a member of the group by lottery for whom we prayed during the program.

The Group

Many of the nurses had prior histories with one another and they quickly generated an atmosphere of trust with open and honest communication. All were female and between forty and sixty-five years old.

Their job descriptions varied considerably. One nurse recently began as the first volunteer parish nurse of a United Methodist congregation. Her large congregation had a history of health ministries, but no parish nurse. During the unit of CPE the congregation offered to increase her position from half-time to full-time in a medical clinic. She continued to volunteer as a parish nurse on a more limited basis. Two other nurses from the same United Church of Christ parish were volunteer health ministers. One focused on women's health issues and the other on cross-cultural conversations among African-American, Hispanic, and Caucasian congregations. By the end of the unit, their projects overlapped in a bible study for women sponsored by these congregations. A fourth nurse was a full-time volunteer with health ministry in a Mennonite congregation. She was trying to develop, diversify, and share the leadership for this ministry while she explored other possibilities for ministry. She also visited patients at the hospital with resident CPE chaplains. By doing this she laid the groundwork for the CPE residents doing the same thing with medical students later in the year. A fifth nurse became a United Methodist Deacon and developed her parish nurse program with a grant from the denomination. She had already developed several screening programs, a healthy lunch program, and a healing service for her congregation. The sixth nurse was employed by the congregation in which she grew up. Her parish nurse program was maturing and trying to involve more people in the congregation. The final nurse had completed a previous CPE unit and was working twenty hours per week at an Episcopal cathedral where she functioned primarily as a health advocate for parishioners involved in the health care system. Many of these patients were on the fringe of the congregation and she struggled with getting more people involved in the healing ministry.

These students reminded me of CPE groups before it became a seminary or denominational requirement. The nurses had chosen CPE because they wanted the experience; their own agendas were clear. The isolation of their individual work made the group relationships a safe haven and a needed respite. Personal issues were interwoven into the fabric of the group; two nurses lost a parent during the unit and several experienced family problems. Three were wrestling with vocational questions.

Supervisory Adjustments

This was the first time I conducted two introductory CPE units at the same time; the other extended unit met all day on Mondays. I felt time constraints during the first few weeks of the program because I visited the clinical sites (parishes) in addition to leading the class times. Starting at 9:00 a.m. was also significant because it gave me time to report with our regular CPE residents and copy material for the parish nurse program.

Since I knew I would have to perform fourteen evaluations for the two CPE programs within the space of one month, I took notes or put vignettes into the final evaluation form on my computer.

Many of the didactics were identical to or modifications of ones I had already done for previous CPE groups or continuing education programs for pastors. It was helpful that I had done previous reading in congregational dynamics because that turned out to be an important topic for the parish nurses.

Personally, I found this unit to be very energizing. In supervision, didactics, and verbatims, I made a concerted effort to focus on spiritual dynamics at the request of the nurses. When I focused too intently on spiritual issues, the nurses reminded me that "sometimes a visit is just a visit."

ISSUES RAISED BY PARISH NURSES

The nurses generally found it helpful to write their autobiography, to complete the Myers-Briggs Type Indicator, the Kolb Learning Style Inventory, and the measuring psychosocial development instruments. It helped them to identify their own personal dynamics and to pull together previously unrelated issues in their lives. Three themes from their CPE experience follow.

Identity and Role

The group process involved several developmental stages. During the first few weeks, the nurses raised identity issues and their practical desire to "fix it"—no matter what "it" was. For some, identity issues arose because this was a new role for them. For others the issue was a desire to change the role because it had grown beyond any reasonable ability to fulfill it. Struggling with the desire to "fix it" provoked discussions of personal limits and the appropriateness of boundaries.

The second area that received attention was how to gain credibility within their congregations. Sometimes this was an issue because fellow volunteers were jealous. For others, it required an examination of their expectations about program growth. This issue often surfaced through the parish nurses' anger or guilt when expectations were not met.

The third area was negotiating their role with other professional church staff, particularly the clergy. Most clergy were supportive, although some were hostile. Others were initially supportive and then became more hesitant. For the nurses who had already negotiated this relationship, their focus was more on navigating transitions in the growth of their programs. For example, one student got in touch with her growing resentment because she was being stretched beyond her own resources. A plan was developed to build a team to make a transition from a more charismatic-leader-centered program to one in which several leaders were responsible for different aspects of the program.

Congregational Dynamics

Concern about congregational dynamics was an increasing focus toward the end of the CPE unit, as the nurses became aware that long-standing congregational struggles were expressing themselves in the parish nurse programs. This issue often appeared as an impasse for the students. They often knew their goals but could not strategize about helpful responses.

Spiritual Dynamics

As mentioned earlier, the unit contained an intentional focus on spiritual issues and how they were interwoven into everyday events. Initial concerns were with spiritual issues confronting their parishioners, some of whom were marginal to congregational life. Other nurses learned how to raise and address spiritual issues with parishioners intimately involved in their congregation.

By midterm, the spiritual issues and practices of the parish nurses themselves came under self-scrutiny. They examined stereotypes of what a devotional life should look like; acknowledged their disappointment with God, the church, or themselves; and experimented with new forms of worship or expressions of devotion.

EVALUATION OF THE PROGRAM

From the Students' Perspectives

In response to the final evaluation question "How has CPE contributed to your understanding of being a parish nurse?" one student wrote:

> CPE brought alive for me the spiritual dimension in parish nursing. CPE has increased my knowledge of the use of scripture in many situations, which before I would have felt uncomfortable using. The course validated for me what I felt was important all along, but was unable or perhaps afraid to put into practice. It feels as if a missing piece has been found. Because I have gained a better understanding of myself, I have been able to broaden my horizons. I am better able to be a presence, a listener and a teacher in my own congregation and with members of the congregation that are different in race and religious interpretation. I am able to be a better listener rather than an advisor in my family.

Another wrote:

> What an enriching experience this has been! The teaching, the resources, the fellowship, the verbatims, and the knowledge of things I knew little of, such as church government and structure, and dynamics. The shared experiences. The caring attitudes. The reminders that God is in all that we do.

A third student wrote, "All of the learning through CPE gives me greater ability to listen, understand, accept, teach, love, lead, and care. Spirituality is the core of health and wholeness."

A fourth student wrote:

> I think the first contribution the program has offered is to realize the need for further learning about the dynamics of people, relationships, family and congregation. As I grow in the knowledge in these areas I will be able to function more effectively as a parish nurse. . . . The verbatim has been a very positive help. It is a step-by-step process of considering all the factors involved in a situation. For me it is a way to step back from the situation and take a better look at it. . . . We talked several times about "being there," that is, being present physically, spiritually or emotionally. CPE has contributed to my understanding of the importance of what that means.

Another student wrote:

> The function of pastoral care as parish nurse has been heightened. But even more so was the interchange between the nurses concerning the situations and problems encountered in their respective church ministries. It helped to put into perspective my own observations and difficulties. . . . More than once I found the topic presented or the subject we were dealing with to be very timely to a situation I was encountering at the time. That is my view of Divine Providence.

The sixth student wrote:

> Documentation can help me in my movement beyond analysis to more depth in theological reflection, planning and follow through. I am learning to understand and appreciate the "foreign" culture and society in which I am functioning. This includes its language, mores, history, politics, structure and how my functioning, values etc are a "foreign" culture to them. I learned how to "marry" the two in a way that caused us to love and know God and His Son and care for each other and not let the differences and externals separate us. Parish nursing is as much pastoral care as it is professional nursing and integrating them as one is a long spiritual/conversion process for myself as well as for the parishioners/staff . . . so be patient! The most effective tool I have to offer is myself, therefore self-development

and self-care is something I need desperately to cultivate both personally and through others. God is building His church and redeeming the world. That is not my job. He has called me to participate faithfully in it but it is not my responsibility.

Most of the students' critiques of the program can be seen in the changes to the content of the didactics. A comparison of the originally proposed curriculum and the final curriculum are illustrated in Table 6.2. Four of the six students returned the standard ACPE participant response form, which asks students to rate eighteen different aspects of the program on a one (very negative) to five (very positive) scale. Of the responses 68 percent rated aspects of the program as "very positive," and 23 percent, as "positive." Only two responses (4 percent) rated the experience as neutral: "This unit of CPE helped me to make optimum use of theology," and "This unit of COPE gave me adequate opportunity to be involved in interdisciplinary relationships in the clinical setting." One student marked this item as "not applicable."

From the Supervisor's Perspective

My own reflections fall into four categories. The first response is joy. This unit was a real delight. The nurses wanted CPE, knew their personal and professional issues, and were willing to discuss them. The curriculum addressed their immediate needs and concerns. I learned a lot about the struggles of parish nursing as a growing movement within the church.

Second, I experienced concerns about how CPE can be adapted to the needs of parish nurses. The CPE standards are written for professional development of clergy. While the current standards are important, they do not fit the role of parish nurse as neatly as the role of chaplain or ordained clergy. When the nurses read the standards they often had different understandings of them than intended by ACPE. With more and more nonordained persons seeking CPE, ACPE will have to address this issue.

Third, I am concerned about a parish pastor wanting to complete CPE and getting credit for work in the parish. Permitting this would deplete our "staff"(students) available for hospital on-call duties. On-call activities are considerable in this institution, and having fewer students would be a problem.

TABLE 6.2. The Proposed and Renegotiated CPE Curricula for Parish Nurses

Week	Proposed Curriculum	Renegotiated Curriculum
1	Learning Contract	
2	Listening Skills	
3	The Sender	
4	The Receiver: Counseling Response	Coping with Unresponsive Patients
5	Crisis Intervention Verbatim	Tacit Contracts and Counseling Responses
6	Stress, Change, and Self-Care	Congregation Health Conference
7	Systems Theory	Stress/Change and Systems Theory
8	Anxiety	Anxiety and Systems Theory
9	Life Cycle	
10	Family Life Cycle	
11	Genogram	Spiritual Diagnosis
12	Parish Dynamics and Rumors	Parish Dynamics
13	Midterm Evaluations	Enneagram completed
14	Negotiating Role	The Elderly
15	Spiritual Assessment	(Snow Day)
16	Substance Abuse	Rumors and Dealing with Rumors
17	Suicide	Anger
18	Depression/Loneliness	Conflict Management
19	Aging	Referrals
20	Dying, Grief, and Loss	Spiritual Assessment
21	Spiritual Interventions I	Tools of Wellness
22	Spiritual Interventions II	Spiritual Interventions
23	Community Resources	Motivation
24	Congregational Assessment and Program Development	Focus on Children
25	Final Evaluations/Graduation	Miracles
26	Final Evaluations/Graduation	

Fourth, the program connected me with other centers that are conducting CPE for parish nurses. Programs exist in Iowa, Tennessee, Illinois, Indiana, and Manitoba, Canada. Other programs likely exist as well. It will clearly be beneficial for such programs to share experiences in the future and to explore the implications of their efforts with the broader CPE movements, both in the United States and Canada.

CONCLUSION

George Fitchett (1999) lists several trends for chaplaincy of the future. He writes, "Chaplains will have the opportunity to address the new and growing emphasis on health and wellness in the community . . . [and] opportunities will increase for chaplains to collaborate with congregations as wellness is encouraged and supported at this grass roots level" (p. 1). This CPE unit with parish nurses allowed me to step into that future, and it was exciting.

REFERENCES

Erikson, Erik (1963). Eight ages of man. In *Childhood and society* (pp. 247-274). New York: W.W. Norton and Co.

Fitchett, George (1999). *The APC News.* Chicago: The Association of Professional Chaplains, March/April.

Gilligan, Carol (1982). *In a different voice.* Cambridge, MA: Harvard University Press.

Pruyser, Paul (1976). Guidelines for pastoral diagnosis. In *Minister as diagnostician* (pp. 60-79). Philadelphia, PA: Westminster Press.

Standards of the Association for Clinical Pastoral Education, Inc. (2000). Decatur, GA. <www.ACPE.edu>.

Chapter 7

A Partnership That Matters: Collaborative Interdisciplinary Ministry Among Faith Community Nurses and Faith Group Leaders

Margaret B. Clark
Joanne K. Olson

The exciting venture known as "parish nursing" began with professional linkages between community nurses and the Pastoral Care Department at Lutheran General Hospital in Park Ridge, Illinois (Westberg, 1987). This health care innovation, of local faith communities hiring registered professional nurses to carry forward an intentional health promotion ministry, is fast contributing to valued partnerships in the provision of health care services around the globe. With such a positive development under way (Solari-Twadell and McDermott, 1999), the time is right for nurses and chaplains to reflect together on models of collaboration that contribute to parish nursing.

This chapter describes how learning across the disciplines of nursing and theology can advance parish nurse education and contribute to professional practice. Our reflections are rooted in experiences we have shared while developing two university nursing courses, an extended unit of clinical pastoral education (CPE) for parish nurses, and while co-authoring a book titled *Nursing Within a Faith Community: Promoting Health in Times of Transition* (Clark and Olson, 2000). In addition, we have "walked beside" numerous faith communities as they have initiated parish nurse ministries. The educational background of the senior author is in theology, and her ministry experi-

89

ences as a CPE supervisor have been in parish-based pastoral care and hospital chaplaincy. The second author is educated in nursing, and her professional interests are in the areas of community and family health, nursing education, nurse-client interaction, spiritual aspects of nursing care, and faith community nursing.[1]

Although we come from different professional backgrounds, we have discovered in our work together a shared affinity for asking questions that are in the service of learning. Indeed, the idea of learning through inquiry appears in both nursing and CPE literature (Boisen, 1945; Gros and Ezer, 1997). It is a questioning approach that can foster health promotion by nurses (Allen, 1986) and faith renewal by pastoral care providers (Groome, 1991). What we share in these pages is interdisciplinary reflection emanating from a "learning through inquiry" approach. In particular, we draw on elements within the McGill model of nursing (Gottlieb and Ezer, 1997) as a framework for use by both nursing-prepared and theologically prepared professionals in advancing ministry collaboration between faith community nurses and faith group leaders. Although the McGill model is as yet little known outside Canada, we hope its core components of "health, family, learning, and collaboration" (Kravitz and Frey, 1989, p. 319) can become better appreciated, and that the model's potential to advance interdisciplinary ministry collaboration can be shared more broadly.

WHAT OUR EXPERIENCE HAS TAUGHT US

We have been working together for approximately five years, in which time we have experienced a maturing awareness of how complementary differences between nursing-prepared and theologically prepared professionals in ministry can contribute to at least three core values related to parish nursing. These values are (1) appreciating holistic linkages between faith and health, (2) exploring interdisciplinary ministry collaboration as a dimension of professional functioning, and (3) envisioning local faith communities as "community health centers" where faith seeking and health seeking are encouraged and wholeness is fostered. We now examine each of these values more closely.

Appreciating Holistic Linkages Between Faith and Health

Every academic discipline and profession has its own terminology or jargon. Thus, when a nurse uses the abbreviation "BP," others need to know that this refers to blood pressure and not British Petroleum. Likewise, when those in the field of theology use terms such as "practical" or "systematic," others need to know that each refers to a field of study within theology and not to a need to be more organized. In the area of faith community nursing, members of one profession enter into professional working relationships with members of another profession. Thus, faith community nurses and theologically educated pastoral leaders need to learn from one another about the academic disciplines and professional languages that inform their respective functioning.

Professionally prepared nurses working within faith community settings are not seeking to replace other ministry professionals or duplicate the functions of other faith group leaders. Rather, the unique role of faith community nurses is to carry forward an intentional health promotion ministry. They foster linkages of health and faith by translating "the language of science and the language of religion" in ways that are helpful to a "whole person" approach to health care (Westberg, 1990a, p. 28). Achieving greater depth of communication in matters of faith and health involves using terminology drawn from both theology and the health sciences. In this regard, parish nurses benefit from learning more about basic theological terminology and the fundamental concepts related to religious/faith traditions. Likewise, faith group leaders benefit from learning more about the health sciences and fundamental health care concepts. What the present authors have learned through experience is that familiarity with each other's professional language enables a climate of dialogue in which linkages between faith and health are appreciated more clearly and communicated more effectively.

Exploring Interdisciplinary Ministry Collaboration

Collaboration among professional disciplines is a growing phenomenon in health care (Seaburn et al., 1996; Sullivan, 1998). Likewise, the idea of "collaboration" is found in the literature of both ministry in general and parish nurse ministry in particular (Lloyd and

Ludwig-Beymer, 1999; Sofield and Juliano, 1987). What does it mean, then, to explore interdisciplinary ministry collaboration between nursing-prepared and theologically prepared professionals who seek further education as well as professional practice development in the field of parish nursing?

In our experience, the idea of "parish nursing" was met with enthusiasm and its potential as an innovative ministry resource within faith communities was easily recognized. This was followed by reading, research, and shared reflection with additional colleagues on various ways in which nursing education, education for ministry, and parish nurse practice development needed to be interrelated. As communication deepened, the interdisciplinary nature of our endeavors became increasingly significant. This was when "collaborating" became more interesting.

At times we found ourselves "bumping into" unexamined worldviews, paradigms, and filters. In this regard, we understand "filters" to be assumptions, attitudes, values, and beliefs that result from experience and affect, or color, the way we view new experiences.[2] For example, while discussing possible tasks of parish nurses within local congregations, we encountered stereotypes, both those which nurses have of pastoral care providers/chaplains and, in turn, those which chaplains/pastoral care providers hold concerning nurses. In addition, our differing professional backgrounds "filtered" our perceptions of commonly held values, such as spirituality, wholeness, ministry, and health. Indeed, each of us brought into our working relationship a number of beliefs and assumptions that were not immediately apparent. It took experiences of "encountering differences" for these beliefs and assumptions to become more visible. Once visible, they could be explored. This is where we discovered that we could make "a decision to learn" (Pierce, Wagner, and Page, 1998, p. 39) across our differences by promoting "inquiry."

Processes of inquiry usually occurred spontaneously. We might be talking about ministry experiences shared by parish nurses in one of our classes. In the course of our conversation, differences of perception might become apparent. For example, both nurses and chaplains are educated in how to respond to those who are newly bereaved. Each professional enters the caring relationship, however, with attention focused on specific assessment concerns. Noticing differences

between nurses and chaplains in assessing needs of the newly bereaved can be an opportunity for interdisciplinary dialogue and collaboration. Such dialogue might begin with asking some open-ended
questions about the other's professional perceptions. For example,
the chaplain author might ask, "As a theologically educated person,
how do you see it?" Or the nurse author might ask, "From a nursing
point of view, what would you suggest?" With exploratory inquiry
comes the sharing of differing worldviews, paradigms, and filters.
Likewise, with ongoing interdisciplinary dialogue, a deeper appreciation of the level of skill and ability each professional brings to a ministry experience can develop. In our experience, this leads to increased colleagueship, shared ministry, mutual empowerment, and
creative planning.

Envisioning Local Faith Communities
As "Community Health Centers"

In keeping with similar practices described by Westberg (1990b,
1999) and Droege (1995), the nurse author often begins presentations
to local congregations with a three-part inquiry. Participants are
asked to name five health care agencies in their community, to indicate whether their local faith community was included on their list,
and to reflect on their rationale for including or not including their
faith community as a health agency (Olson, 2000). Over time she has
observed that agencies commonly identified include the nearest hospital, a dental office, a physician's office, or a neighborhood walk-in
clinic. While there are no right or wrong answers to the inquiry, discussions that follow the questioning are quite informative. They reveal much about how the group views health and which community
agencies provide health care according to the participants' definitions
of health. Finally, this leads to a consideration of what health is and
why faith communities might be considered "community health centers" and vital partners in the provision of community health care.

As "health" becomes an increasingly relevant topic in all circles of
society, so it is becoming a topic of conversation in local parishes,
temples, and synagogues. In this regard, greater emphasis is being
given to local congregations as places of initial contact with the
health care system. This is the domain of primary health care and a
natural locus for health promotion. Health promotion, the type that

enables people to increase control over and improve their health (World Health Organization, Health and Welfare Canada, and Canadian Public Health Association, 1986), can be significantly advanced by means of the health services identified with parish nurse ministry (Holstrom, 1999). That is to say, health education, confidential health counseling, health referral, developing support groups, health advocacy, facilitating awareness of faith-health linkages, and recruiting, training, as well as supervising volunteer health workers are ministry processes that enable people to increase control over and improve their health. We are convinced that local congregations offer a natural, circumscribed environment for implementing principles of primary health care and evaluating outcomes related to health issues arising among individuals, families, and groups. With more attention given to faith communities as one of the points at which health services are mobilized and coordinated, local congregations will become increasingly recognized as health-promoting, illness-preventing care providers who manage ongoing health problems (Provincial Health Council of Alberta, 1997). Likewise, local faith communities will be more readily viewed as partners in the full spectrum of healing, health, wholeness, and health promotion.

THE MCGILL MODEL OF NURSING INFORMS OUR COLLABORATIVE EXPERIENCE

As educators, we value learning. In our interdisciplinary work related to parish nurse course and practice development, learning has fueled our efforts and focused our attention. Imagine how exciting it was for the pastoral education author to hear about a nursing model that included among its core components the value of learning! Further, imagine how enthusiastic both authors became as they discovered the interdisciplinary potential in drawing upon this nursing model as a dimension of their collaborative ministry! How did this model become so important to us? Much of it has to do with "five broad questions" that are available through the McGill model of nursing (Allen, 1986). We believe these questions frame a tripartite reflective process with potential to guide not only nurses but also faith group leaders and clients/congregants in "learning through inquiry" about both health and faith (Clark and Olson, 2000). We shall return to these questions shortly. Before we do, however, a few words about McGill's nursing approach are necessary.

The McGill model of nursing was developed by Moyra Allen and other faculty at the McGill School of Nursing, McGill University, Montreal, Quebec, Canada. Impetus for the model's development grew largely out of changes in Canada's health care system in the early 1960s when health care services became universally available to all Canadians. With the thought that nursing would play a major role in the restructured health system, debate occurred regarding what the nursing role would encompass. Rather than expanding the nurses' role into the medical domain, Allen envisioned nurses functioning in a "complemental role" insofar as they possess knowledge and skills that are different from and complementary to physicians and other professionals (Allen, 1977). Furthermore, Allen envisioned a healthier society brought about through the health promotion activities of nurses collaborating with individuals and families. The model she developed addresses ways of mobilizing community resources that empower the healthy development of families throughout their life spans (Allen, 1983). In this model, nurses assume a collaborative relationship with individuals, families, and groups to foster optimal learning in matters of health and health promotion. Although in-depth discussion on the McGill model is beyond the scope of this chapter, many references of relevance to its development occur in the volume by Gottlieb and Ezer (1997).

Returning to the five questions of the McGill model referred to earlier, we reiterate the value of "questioning" as one that is held by both theologically educated and nursing-educated ministry professionals (Gros and Ezer, 1997; Schillebeeckx, 1984). Likewise, we recognize that in matters of both health and faith, inquiry is linked with a process of learning (Allen, 1986; Dulles, 1994). The specific guiding questions provided by Allen are the following:

1. What is the family working on or dealing with?
2. How is the family going about it?
3. What does the family want or what is it working toward?
4. What resources are the family using and what other resources could be mobilized?
5. What aspects of the broader context of family life might explain the family's present health behavior or situation? (Allen, 1986)

These questions consider people within the context of community. The "client," therefore, is always communal in nature. This is true whether working with an individual, family, or group. While not intended by Allen, this approach is congruous with faith, spirituality, theology, religion, health, and health promotion as concepts wherein connections to community are integrally related with personal wholeness and/or wellness (Clark and Olson, in press).

What we suggest is that, by means of Allen's questions, faith community nurses and faith group leaders can participate in a learning dialogue with their clients/congregants that promotes inquiry into matters of both faith and health. Thus, in asking the question "What is the client dealing with?" we expect nurses to identify health issues and faith group leaders to explore faith issues. Likewise, when asking about "resources" we expect nurses to draw upon their knowledge of health resources and religious leaders to access a wealth of faith resources. However, it is in the learning dialogue of client, faith community nurse, and faith group leader that something "new" starts to happen. That is, through collaborative learning with clients/congregants, both nurses and faith group leaders start to explore ways that health issues and faith issues are "connecting" for the client. Here new questions may arise to confirm, expand upon, and/or reframe the congregant's deepening level of awareness. Increased consciousness, in turn, cycles back through the shared learning process to new points of connection, further questioning, deepened awareness, and so forth. Some examples of new questions that can arise out of this kind of collaborative learning are the following: Where is there evidence of "wholeness" as the client engages in health-seeking activities that may start to relate with the client's faith seeking? How can faith resources and health resources complement each other in supporting and empowering this client/congregant? How can spiritual/religious resources within the unique heritage of this particular faith community provide a context for health promotion that sheds light on the client's present health situation? We now turn from these rather abstract considerations to something more practical and grounded in ministry experience.

COLLABORATIVE LEARNING THROUGH INQUIRY

In the following vignette we examine a ministry experience[3] involving collaborative learning through inquiry among a congregant family, faith community nurse, and faith group leader. First we present a narrative that introduces the health situation affecting the "Miller family." Following this, one of the five guiding questions from the McGill model (#4: What resources are the family using and what other resources could be mobilized?) is used to frame inquiry by the pastoral leader and parish nurse. Their questioning facilitates assessment and collaborative reflection with the Millers. Out of this shared ministry approach, points of connection occur and a learning dialogue gives rise to new questions. These are the places where health promotion and faith renewal "connect" for the Millers, empowering them to achieve improved health and wholeness. Although space constraints prevent us from developing all five of the McGill questions in relationship with this ministry vignette, the reader can gain a sense of the process.

A Ministry Vignette

Darrel Miller works as a city planner.[4] His wife, Louise, a textile fabric designer, delivered their second child two weeks ago. Soon after the birth a number of concerns were raised regarding baby Matthew's health, and it was subsequently determined that their son has Down's syndrome. News of this congenital condition came as a shock to both Darrel and Louise, and they have been unable to make sense of it. Furthermore, since Darrel believed that it is a man's gene which carries the condition, he began to feel guilty and blame himself. Since Darrel is a religious man with many links to the church, he turned to his faith community for support. After talking over his sense of guilt and self-blame with Pastor Martin he felt some relief. He was especially impressed by the pastor's ability to listen to his mixed-up words, thoughts, and occasional emotional outbursts. He was encouraged when Pastor Martin told him about a nurse who was working in the parish to support people at such times as this. With the understanding that his wife was agnostic and may not be comfortable with church-related outreach, Darrel gave the pastor permission to talk with the faith community nurse about their baby's condition. Several evenings later, after talking by telephone with both Darrel and Louise, Katherine, the faith community nurse, came to their home for an initial visit. Katherine prepared for the meeting with Darrel and Louise by familiarizing herself with details of the baby's medical condition, compiling a list of local resources as well as support networks for parents with Down's syndrome children, and consulting with Pastor Martin regarding his ongoing involvement. In the course of her first meeting with Darrel and Louise Miller, Katherine was able to draw on a great deal of the collected information. Her approach, however, was open-ended, and this made both Louise and Darrel feel as if they were intimately involved in every aspect of the discussion.

Guiding Question #4—What Resources Are the Family Using, and What Other Resources Could be Mobilized?

Exploring "Health" Resources

When meeting with Louise and Darrel, the faith community nurse offered a number of possible resources that they had not considered as they tried to learn how to live with their son having Down's syndrome. The couple was unaware, for example, that at least one other couple in the congregation had a child with Down's syndrome. They were unaware, as well, of the early childhood education programs available within the community for children with Down's syndrome. Regarding planning for future children, Louise and Darrel expressed much fear and concern and had some misinformation regarding the congenital nature of Down's syndrome. They were not aware of the excellent genetic counseling services available at the local university hospital. Finally, the couple was unaware of the support groups available to parents with children who have genetic abnormalities. The faith community nurse was able to assist the family in accessing the resources that they decided to seek out and to "walk beside them" as they made difficult decisions about whether to have more children.

Exploring Faith Resources

Darrel's initial recourse to his faith community was for crisis intervention. His guilt and shame prevented him from relating with both Louise and his new son, Matthew. After coming through that crisis he was open to ongoing contact with his faith community through meetings with the faith community nurse, Katherine. It was in this relationship that additional faith resources opened up for both Darrel and Louise. For years Darrel had practiced his religion alone. Likewise, he and Louise had an understanding that the children could attend church with Darrel but would not be formally initiated until they were adults and could make their own choice. As a nurse, Katherine posed no threat to Louise's sensitivity regarding religion. Although Katherine was from Darrel's faith community, Louise saw her strictly as a health care worker. As the relationship developed, opportunities arose to celebrate special health-related events in Matthew's life. Some of these were rites of passage, others were achievements, and still others addressed feelings of discouragement or fatigue. At first Katherine offered, and then was regularly asked, to lead the rituals honoring these events. As the value of ritual grew for this family, they found a number of ways to create and participate in events that took Matthew into the broader community. Thus, they regularly attended parades, public ceremonies, treasure hunts, and similar activities. In these ways, rituals contributed to Matthew's widening social integration and to the family's ability to face both good times and bad in a spirit of solidarity.

Points of Connection and Deepening
in Collaborative Learning

In light of Matthew's health condition of Down's syndrome, Pastor Martin and Katherine knew that a long-term process of accompaniment would be necessary. With Darrel and Louise's permission they began to involve the broader faith community in supportive ways. First, they saw a need to educate the congregation regarding the abilities as well as limitations experienced by those with Down's syndrome. Darrel and Louise met the other couple in the faith community who had a Down's syndrome child. This child's parents and Darrel decided to bring their children with them to church, just as Darrel was in the habit of doing with his other child. The modeling of the two families stimulated a wonderful response of inclusiveness among other members of the congregation. They were touched by the loving presence communicated by these two young people with Down's syndrome. They became valued members of the faith community and contributed to its mission of outreach. Katherine included this sense of Matthew's outreach role in her ritual connections with the family.

As Matthew matured, his family found ways for him to "go to school" and/or "go to work." That is, anytime he was discovering some new task or capability, they called it school. They also acknowledged Matthew's capacity to express love and affection as a strength that was parallel to a job skill. When Matthew was asked to take a turn cuddling infants in the congregation's day care center, he said he was going to work with his "loving skills."

At times through the years Darrel, Louise, and their family experienced doubt, discouragement, and frustration. They wrestled with the questions "Why did this congenital condition occur in our family?" and "Why do *we* have a child with a condition that asks so much of us all the time?" In this regard, both Katherine and Pastor Martin accompanied them, suggesting resources for self-care and family support. On one occasion, Pastor Martin told them about the writings of Jean Vanier and the L'Arche communities he founded.[5] The belief within these communities is that people with limited mental abilities have something special to teach us. In particular, they have something to teach us about what it means to "love" and "be loved." Learning more about Vanier as well as L'Arche opened both Darrel and Louise to a sort of spiritual bond that was new for them. They read and discussed the writings of Vanier and others affected by the L'Arche philosophy. In its own peculiar way, the questioning process carried forward by the Miller family over the course of many years enabled faithfulness and respect to be the mainstay in parenting Matthew. Having access to the collaborative support of Katherine and Pastor Martin, as well as the inclusive consciousness of Darrel's faith community, gave them deep grounding in their faith-health integration.

CONCLUDING REMARKS

With the advent of a new millennium it is important to respect what has gone before. This is true not only in the realms of nursing and chaplaincy but also for the historic relationship between faith and health. What better way to respect their interconnected past than by having faith group leaders and parish/faith community nurses engage in collaborative learning through inquiry? Indeed, gaining familiarity with the differing knowledge bases, professional languages, values, assumptions, and filtering processes that inform our unique professions promises significant benefit for all involved. Likewise, drawing upon theoretical frameworks that foster interdisciplinary ministry collaboration can empower those being served to think inclusively and act in ways that integrate both health promotion and faith renewal. In this vein, our experience with the McGill model of nursing to guide collaborative learning in ministry is something we offer in support of parish nursing education and practice development.

NOTES

1. Throughout this chapter we broaden the concepts of "parish nursing" and "parish" by using "faith community nurse" and "faith community" in order to include the rich diversity of faith traditions existing in our world.

2. This definition of "filters" grew out of a discussion with participants of the University of Alberta Faculty of Nursing's 1999 summer theory course, "Nursing 498: Promoting Well-Being in Faith Communities."

3. The ministry experience described in this chapter is an amalgamation of several events. Names and identifying circumstances of those originally involved have been altered to preserve confidentiality.

4. This narrative is based on one of six ministry vignettes developed in our book (Clark and Olson, 2000). In that text, four chapters are dedicated to in-depth reflection on a faith community nurse's use of the McGill nursing model with the "Brown family." Later, after developing our thoughts on the interdisciplinary ministry potential within the McGill approach, an additional chapter was dedicated to sharing five faith community ministry narratives, with special emphasis given to each of the five McGill questions.

5. L'Arche is an international federation of communities in which people with developmental disabilities and their assistants live, work, pray, and share their lives together. Founded in 1964 by Jean Vanier and Father Thomas Philippe in France, over 100 L'Arche communities exist around the world at present. See the Web page <http://www.dsuper.net/~jcpas/aaccueil.html> for more information.

REFERENCES

Allen, M. (1977). Comparative theories of the expanded role in nursing and implications for nursing practice: A working paper. *Nursing Papers, 9*(2), 38-45.

Allen, M. (1986). A developmental health model: Nursing as continuous inquiry. In *Nursing theory congress: Theoretical pluralism: Directions for a practice discipline* [Cassette recording]. Markham, Ontario, Canada: Audio Archives of Canada.

Allen, M. (1997). Primary care nursing: Research in action. In L. Gottlieb and H. Ezer (Eds.), *A perspective on health, family, learning and collaborative nursing: A collection of writings on the McGill model of nursing* (pp. 164-190). Montreal, Quebec, Canada: McGill University School of Nursing.

Boisen, A. (1945). Cooperative inquiry in religion. In G. Asquith (Ed.), *Vision from a little known country: A Boisen reader* (pp. 77-87). Decatur, GA: Journal of Pastoral Care Publications.

Clark, M. and Olson, J. (2000). *Nursing within a faith community: Promoting health in times of transition.* Thousand Oaks, CA: Sage Publications.

Droege, T.A. (1995). Congregations as communities of health and healing. *Interpretations: A Journal of Bible and Theology, 49*(2), 117-129.

Dulles, A. (1994). *The assurance of things hoped for.* New York: Oxford University.

Gottlieb, L. and Ezer, H. (1997). *A* perspective on health, family, learning, and collaborative nursing: A collection of writings on the McGill model of nursing. Montreal, Quebec, Canada: McGill University School of Nursing.

Groome, T. (1991). *Sharing faith.* New York: Harper-Collins.

Gros, C. and Ezer, H. (1997). Promoting inquiry and nurse-client collaboration: A unique approach to teaching and learning. In L. Gottlieb and H. Ezer (Eds.), *A perspective on health, family, learning and collaborative nursing: A collection of writings on the McGill model of nursing* (pp. 219-225). Montreal, Quebec, Canada: McGill University School of Nursing.

Holstrom, S. (1999). Perspectives on a suburban parish nursing practice. In P.A. Solari-Twadell and M.A. McDermott (Eds.), *Parish nursing: Promoting whole person health within faith communities* (pp. 67-74). Thousand Oaks, CA: Sage Publications.

Kravitz, M. and Frey, M. (1989). The Allen nursing model. In J. Fitzpatrick and A. Whall (Eds.), *Conceptual models of nursing: Analysis and application* (pp. 313-329). Norwalk, CT: Appleton and Lange, 313-329.

Lloyd, R. and Ludwig-Beymer, P. (1999). Listening to faith communities: Collaboration with those served. In P.A. Solari-Twadell and M. McDermott (Eds.), *Parish nursing: Promoting whole person health within faith communities* (pp. 107-121). Thousand Oaks, CA: Sage Publications.

Olson, J. (2000). Health, healing, wholeness, and health promotion. In M. Clark and J. Olson (Eds.), *Nursing within a faith community: Promoting health in times of transition.* Thousand Oaks, CA: Sage Publications.

Pierce, C., Wagner, D., and Page, B. (1998). *A male/female continuum: Paths to colleagueship,* Expanded edition. Laconia, NH: New Dynamics Publications.

Provincial Health Council of Alberta (1997). *Provincial Health Council of Alberta 1997 Annual Report: Primary Health System.* Edmonton, Alberta, Canada: Alberta Health and Wellness.

Schillebeeckx, E. (1984). *The Schillebeeckx reader.* New York: Crossroad.

Seaburn, D., Lorenz, A., Gunn, W., Gawinski, B., and Mauksch, L. (1996). *Models of collaboration.* New York: Basic Books.

Sofield, L. and Juliano, C. (1987). *Collaborative ministry.* Notre Dame, IN: Ave Maria Press.

Solari-Twadell, P. and McDermott, M. (Eds.) (1999). *Parish nursing: Promoting whole person health within faith communities.* Thousand Oaks, CA: Sage Publications.

Sullivan, T. (1998). *Collaboration: A health care imperative.* New York: McGraw-Hill.

Westberg, G. (1987). *The parish nurse: How to start a parish nurse program in your church.* Park Ridge, IL: Parish Nurse Resource Center.

Westberg, G. (1990a). A historical perspective: Wholistic health and the parish nurse. In P.A. Solari-Twadell, A.M. Djupe, and M.A. McDermott (Eds.), *Parish nursing: The developing practice* (pp. 27-39). Park Ridge, IL: National Parish Nurse Resource Center.

Westberg, G. (1990b). *The parish nurse: Providing a minister of health for your congregation.* Minneapolis, MN: Augsburg Fortress.

Westberg, G.E. (1999). A personal historical perspective of whole person health and the congregation. In P.A. Solari-Twadell and M.A. McDermott (Eds.), *Parish nursing: Promoting whole person health within faith communities* (pp. 35-41). Thousand Oaks, CA: Sage Publications.

World Health Organization, Health and Welfare Canada, and Canadian Public Health Association (1986). Ottawa charter for health promotion. Ottawa, Ontario: Canada Health and Welfare.

Chapter 8

Nurses and the Clergy Working Together: Meeting the Challenge

Joan L. Murray
Dawn B. Rigney

BACKGROUND

Educators must help parish nurses integrate their professional contribution into congregational settings. This integration process is unique for each congregation and each nurse because it involves the individual nurse's relationship with God. Thus, the ministry of parish nursing is influenced by the degree to which each nurse integrates his or her spiritual life into the practice of nursing.

Theological and nursing educators must work together to facilitate this integration even though they stand within different professions. These theological and nursing educators must do their homework together. They must understand their own spiritual lives and integrate them into ministry and professional practice. This encourages them to talk with one another as they develop health ministry education programs.

In this chapter the authors describe the challenge of integrating their two professional perspectives into a health ministry institute for the purpose of preparing parish nurses. At the very beginning, problems emerged when the theological educator kept using terms such as "embrace" and the nurse educator insisted on setting goals and objectives as the first step. Differences also appeared when discussing the name of the institute; one educator preferred "health ministry" while the other suggested "parish nursing."

Note: A copy of the program is available from the first author.

The four members of the planning committee all possessed nursing credentials, including the theological educator, and were members of the Central Virginia Health Ministry Association. Two were actively pursuing a career in parish nursing and completed the course during this planning process. The challenge to integrate the professions included clarification of knowledge from nursing, theology, pastoral care, adult education, and parish nursing. The first step was to build working relationships.

RELATIONSHIP BUILDING

We met regularly to plan the institute and allowed extra time for sharing and prayer as a way to learn about one another. After some experimentation, we deliberately chose a setting that seemed the most conducive to building relationships.

We began by discussing our backgrounds and family histories. Our continued dialogue uncovered similarities in culture, educational background, religion, and interests; two of us discovered immediately that we were from similar towns in West Virginia. We then explored the similarities in our professions. We discussed a deep commitment to the interconnectedness of all aspects of life, including health and illness. The professionals in both disciplines addressed that interconnectedness in their own particular ways. We also discovered our motivation was the same: to prepare nurses for health ministry in congregations.

As a result of these efforts, we established the crucial trust necessary for productive relationships and this provided safety in expressing our opinions and exploring our differences. There were times of tension. For example, on one occasion we were intensely discussing student selection processes. Several of us strongly disagreed but reached an agreement after a couple of meetings. We then learned that the clergy husband of one of our members was praying for us.

As we explored our different opinions, we began to collaborate in developing the curriculum. This was accomplished through understanding, compromising, and negotiating as we learned to appreciate one another's varying viewpoints. We recognized two major differences that impacted the planning process: our individual perceptions of parish nursing and our varied approaches to planning. These differences and their resolution are briefly described here.

PERCEPTIONS OF PARISH NURSING

Since we possessed limited knowledge and experience in parish nursing, we needed to clarify our thinking; it was basic to collaboratively planning the institute. We attended a workshop on parish nursing sponsored by the Central Virginia Health Ministry Association. Our understanding of parish nursing was derived from the content of that workshop, our background readings about parish nursing, and dialogue with other members of the health ministry association. During subsequent planning sessions, therefore, the four team members shared their ideas and understanding of parish nursing as well as their vision for the future of this discipline. Four distinct perceptions and visions emerged. For example, the clergy perceived spirituality as the center of health ministry. The nurse educator envisioned health care as being the primary focus. We also recognized that our differences reflected those we could anticipate in our audience. Acknowledging these differences resulted in compromise.

APPROACH TO PLANNING

We recognized three differences in regard to the planning process:

1. Perception of planning time
2. Ideas for the target audience
3. Focus for the institute

Our collaboration required more time for planning than was anticipated by the nurse educator and the clergy. Nursing educators typically demonstrate highly developed skills for curriculum development including goals and objectives. Spiritual/pastoral care and education professionals are just beginning to appreciate these skills. Much time was given to formulating institute goals and objectives.

The discussion regarding goals and objectives revealed diverse ideas concerning target audiences. For instance, the nurse educator anticipated 150 participants with nationally known speakers. Other team members suggested twenty-five to fifty participants from the community with locally known speakers. We compromised by deciding this would be a pilot project targeting the local community with a maximum of fifty participants and promised another institute program for a larger audience later. Registered nurses were the targeted audience, and we asked local speakers to provide lectures and lead discussions. We decided to offer continuing education units, and, ironically, the publicity we received from this offering resulted in a statewide response.

Having compromised on two key differences, we began to plan the curriculum. We formulated behavioral objectives that met the standards for continuing education credits from the American Nurses Association and the Association of Professional Chaplains. Clearly, we spoke different professional languages and this required compromise when planning the content. For instance, we needed to integrate concepts such as "embrace" into measurable objectives. We utilized education principles by moving from the general to the specific, integrating spiritual/theological perspectives into nursing practice. We started with the spiritual/theology because that language was new to the nurse planners and was anticipated to be new to the audience.

As we identified the content areas and presentation methodologies, we continued to negotiate and compromise. We sought to balance the theoretical, relational, and experiential dimensions of the curriculum for an anticipated audience of varied backgrounds, knowledge, and experience who also likely possessed multiple perceptions and experiences with parish nursing.

Recognizing that we had only thirty hours to present the content, we began setting priorities concerning the components that each discipline regarded as critical. The clergy person was familiar with a core group of individuals from the Health Ministries Association who would participate in the institute. They were in different stages of developing their own health ministry programs. The clergy, therefore, suggested a considerable time allotment for the relational dimension of the curriculum; the focus of the nurse educator was on the theoretical nursing component. During the course of negotiations, the nurse educator was able to reclaim the relational/spiritual dimension of nursing that was the basis for her own nursing education in a diploma school years previously. The context for the practice of a health ministry focused on the relationship between the parish nurse and the congregation, the relationship among members of the congregation, and the individual nurse's relationship with God. We intentionally planned participant meals and breaks together in the same learning space to promote and encourage networking and community building. The result was a balance in the spiritual, psychological, physical, and social dimensions of health as discussed by Solari-Twadell (1999).

THE INSTITUTE PROGRAM

The Parish/Congregational Health Ministry Institute sponsored by the Central Virginia Health Ministry Association, the University of Virginia School of Nursing, and the University of Virginia Health System was held August 9 through 13, 1999, at the School of Nursing. Seventeen registered nurses participated in the institute. Several of the nurses had already developed their health ministry programs. Four nurses represented a health system and were planning to develop their own training programs. The participants came from a variety of areas throughout the state, representing the Christian (Protestant and Catholic), Unitarian Universalist, and Jewish faith traditions. Estimated ages ranged from the thirties to the sixties with diverse ethnic groups and cultures represented. Participants found local accommodations; breakfast and lunch were provided to promote relationship building. Nursing and religious leaders from the university and surrounding communities spoke and led workshops.

Outcome evaluations indicated the participants liked the interactive methodology and the relational approach. They responded favorably to the movement from the general to the specific in the curriculum, and the content was well received. Speakers' handouts were made available on a resource table that also included parish resources and health-related materials. We included nurses on the panel who were using a variety of models for their own health ministries. Sixteen of the seventeen participants received full continuing education credits for nursing and/or from the Association for Professional Chaplains. The speakers agreed to make themselves available for consultation after the institute.

Evaluation feedback included the need for more emphasis on legal issues related to health ministry, and a request was made for additional step-by-step help in setting up programs. These are being offered through the Health Ministries Association. Textbooks and readings well in advance of the institute were suggested to facilitate a more comprehensive understanding of the concepts. Speakers and participants felt the institute was a valuable education experience.

In summary, the process of writing this chapter and telling our story helped us realized that our collaboration paralleled the evolution of the parish nurse movement. The movement started from a singular beginning and evolved into a health ministry. A strong connection among those committed to parish nursing will nurture the development of meaningful health ministries within congregations. For this, we are grateful.

REFERENCE

Solari-Twadell, Phyllis A. (1999). The emerging practice of parish nursing. In Solari-Twadell, P. A. and McDermott, M. A. (Eds.), *Parish Nursing: Promoting Whole Person Health Within Faith Communities.* Thousand Oaks, CA: Sage Publications.

SECTION IV:
INTERPROFESSIONAL DYNAMICS

Chapter 9

How to Begin a Parish Health Ministry: A Juggling Act

Joyce Kaatz
Tammy Anderson
Valerie Putnam
Don Lehmann

Most of us have seen good jugglers in action. They put the audience at ease, as the balls magically float through the air. They work in unison, sharing the responsibilities to maintain the balls in a constant, even movement, creating beauty. This juggling act did not come easily because practice, constant communication, and even a few mistakes and dropped balls were necessary. This is a metaphor for parish health ministry. When done well, the clergy, nurse, and, in some situations, the chaplain need to interact carefully because parish health ministry is a shared responsibility.

This chapter addresses issues pertaining to the juggling of the parish health ministry between the parish nurse and clergy with regard to responsibilities, parishioners, and programs. We discuss issues that challenge most health ministry teams and suggest strategies and interventions that address these issues, thus promoting a stronger parish health ministry.

PREJUGGLING

Most jugglers do best while standing firmly on a flat, smooth surface. While it is exciting to see a juggler teetering on a plank or standing on a moving ladder, everyone recognizes the risks of difficulties. Parish nurses, and parish health ministries, likewise have an easier and earlier success when they have the opportunity to start their ministry on a firm foundation. A parish program is almost impossible if key congregational leaders or clergy do not understand, desire, or support it.

Establishing a good foundation can happen in a variety of ways and at a variety of speeds. It may happen quickly when a new clergy comes from a congregation that has experienced an effective parish health ministry or if hard-working congregational leaders enable it to happen. It may also occur slowly, perhaps in a large congregation with its many facets and where the wheels of change move slowly. In these situations, it may take years of one clergy or leader attending conferences, talking, and slowly selling people and committees on the value of parish health ministry. But no matter how it occurs, it is valuable to have someone respected by the congregation as a strong advocate, a champion, to prepare the way for health ministry.

It is interesting to note how even God did not just "send His Son," but he sent John the Baptist to prepare the way. How many parish nurses would love to have a John the Baptist to prepare the way for them? Most of us are not that fortunate.

What if you believe that a congregation could benefit from parish health ministry and you want to play a part in getting that ministry started? Although the clergy may not be completely sold on the idea of parish health, they must be at least open to learning about it. Just as a juggler cannot juggle many balls without the support of others, so the parish nurse needs others who express support for the program. Here are some effective steps in selling the program at the beginning:

- Forming groups of health professionals and others interested in health to discuss their thoughts concerning the healing of the body, mind, and soul
- Submitting small articles concerning health and health-related events in the bulletin and monthly newsletter
- Organizing a task force to explore the idea of parish health (eventually these people might be instrumental in starting your health cabinet)
- Providing healing services
- Talking with local hospital chaplains and health systems to discover their ideas
- Visiting other congregations with parish nurses
- Having parish nurses or others committed to parish health ministry speak to the congregation

These months or years of preparation can be most frustrating to those who have "seen the vision" for parish health in a congregation and really want it to start today. The program, however, must go at its own speed, selling its value to all the key players for its eventual success. Without this early nurturing and patience, the program will fail.

ENTERING THE ARENA

Some parish nurses tell stories about failure. Often they entered a congregation, sometimes uninvited, with their own ideas about how a parish health program could be helpful. They met resistance and eventually failed. These churches are actually worse off than before because a new parish nurse program will need to overcome old feelings and biases. How could it have been handled differently?

Parish nurses must enter a congregation as if entering someone's house. In unsuccessful or marginal programs, the difficulties may root in how the nurse entered this new home, the new church family. First, think how you enter a home. As we said before, parish nurses should not just "show up" unannounced; rather, it is better when the people already "living there," the staff and congregational members, know the parish nurse is arriving. We would not just show up and say, "Here I am!" Most people do not like surprises. Instead, we would enter a home politely, humbly, and with caution. We would sit in the living room for a while and watch the family dynamics to assess when to talk and just what kind of family this is. Who is the leader? How do they communicate? Similar to families, church staffs and congregations already have established dynamics. One must determine if this family has many unresolved issues, or whether its members are fairly stable. Will they feel threatened by the nurse, the new person in the family?

We serve best when we wait to be invited to participate, and then sit wherever we are instructed to sit. We need to listen to the hosts' dreams, visions, and thoughts as to our role and then slowly to add our own. Many parish health philosophies suggest that success occurs when we help other people's visions and dreams come true. A parish nurse's dream and passion may be to start nutrition or weight control classes, but if the clergy's main concern is a teenage depression support group, it is best to begin there. While working together in openness to start this new program, the clergy, parish nurse, and parishioners will experience community and success that will lead to other programming efforts. In a new home, we would not enter voicing all our ideas on how to change things and with our own agenda. We would be careful and slow in making changes in the present family agendas and build on what is presently being done. This is not to say parish nurses have to ignore their own visions and dreams. It is all a matter of timing and balance. Enter slowly, listen more than you talk, and follow the lead of family members who have been there before you.

BEGINNING JUGGLING

Back to the arena. First of all, the ringmaster, the clergy, has to be part of the selection process in choosing the nurse. There must be chemistry and an ability to say, "I can work with this person." If a hospital is hiring the nurse, it may initially select a few nurses who would be appropriate for the job, but the church, and especially the clergy, should have the final decision. It is important for the nurse and the clergy to be comfortable with each other's theology.

A ringmaster may come out and announce, "In the center ring we now have the Magnificent Jugglers." The audience sees the jugglers as a team. So it is in health ministry. They are announced and must function as a team, integrated with the parish clergy and hospital chaplain. This is expedited when team members introduce one another at church council, church family nights, as well as informal and planned meetings. Team building can also occur when the clergy and parish nurse connect with area hospital chaplains. As stated previously, most people do not appreciate surprises, so it is important to include chaplains in the vision for parish health ministry. Early and regular dialogue with them as part of the team is important. With the fast-moving changes in hospital systems, hospital chaplains may not be informed when parish nurses begin their ministry. The nurse can organize a meeting with the chaplains to begin to build relationships.

A formal installation service can legitimize a team ministry that includes a parish health program. Such an occasion demonstrates to the congregation that the parish nurse is a partner because the clergy blesses and supports this new ministry. Many installation rituals can be adapted for this occasion and should include congregational responses that commit them to actively supporting this ministry. On the installation weekend, the ritual should be repeated at each worship service.

An amusing thing happened when one program installed their health cabinet. The service was broadcast on television and a viewer saw her retired physician on the cabinet. The viewer called the church in hopes that now her "favorite doctor whom she misses so much" could visit her in her home. In this particular situation that action was not appropriate, but this response from one person does demonstrate that when the path is prepared and the foundation solid and level, people are put at ease. The congregation must recognize this ministry as carried out by a group of professionals working together in parish health.

KEEPING THE BALLS IN THE AIR

Educate, educate, and then educate some more. Juggling does not come easily; it takes hours and days of practice on the part of all the jugglers—and it includes teaching others just what "juggling" is—its beauty and value. In networking with parish nurses, it is amazing and frustrating to hear nurses who complain about always having to answer the question "What does a parish nurse do?" This question is asked often by fellow church staff, parishioners, the general public, and hospital staff. Situations such as these are the perfect opportunity for members of the parish health ministry to describe the roles and goals of the program.

In handling such questions, try this: Thank them for asking; tell them you love to talk about parish ministry (and mean it). Convey that a parish health program involves not only the nurse but also the pastors, other staff, and church volunteers. Keep it short to allow time to hear their thoughts and questions on the topic. Offer to do an adult forum or come to their committee to talk more about parish health.

It may be helpful to develop a handout that can be adapted to discussions and forums from ten to ninety minutes in length. Forums involve group discussion and utilize the same questions used in the team ministry installation to enlist the group's support of the program. Always carry your business card and a brochure (they can be created very inexpensively) so questioners have written information and a means to contact you later. Then allow time for people to share their thoughts and ideas about what you have said and, if possible, discover if they would like to be involved. Some of our best cardiopulmonary resuscitation (CPR) instructors, small support group leaders, and respite care volunteers have emerged from these opportunities to educate and excite others about the ministry.

It is also necessary to provide education for the health ministry team. Attending parish health conferences together will enable the clergy, nurse, cabinet members, and congregational leaders to grow stronger as a team. If conferences are not available or beyond the budget, sponsor an informational event at your church or hospital on "What is parish health?". This ministry is strengthened only when novices and leaders in parish health come together to network and share their stories, journeys, challenges, and dreams.

One of the best resources for the parish nurse is clinical pastoral education (CPE). This national program is provided by medical and parish institutions to help clergy grow in their understanding of themselves and pastoral care. Parish nursing is not a nurse working in the church as a clinical site in which to do nursing. Parish nursing is a commitment to being cross-trained, with skills in both pastoral care and nursing, bringing the two together to enrich both. Parish nursing is an integration of both professions. Therefore, the nurse must be educated, supervised in, and understand the professional ethics of ministry. Usually the primary profession is nursing rather than ministry, and therefore CPE is an excellent educational resource for the nurse. A half unit of CPE each year for parish nurses may be helpful as a way to build professional skills and enhance their integration into ministry. A spiritual counselor can also guide people in health ministry and support spiritual growth.

LOSING CONTROL OF THE BALLS
(EMBRACING CONFLICT)

Most of us would prefer to ignore areas of friction and times when all the balls seem out of control. But just as Job's experience in the Bible, these times of trials can be great times of growth.

Not only must the congregation embrace the concept of parish nursing, but the clergy or pastoral staff must wholeheartedly embrace the concept or it will not work. A major question for the parish nurse and clergy concerns professional boundaries. Boundaries are built on strong relationships with integrity, trust, teamwork, and giftedness. Many areas can cause conflict, as demonstrated in the following parish story. A church with a strong parish nursing program installed a new youth pastor. He had never heard of parish nursing, did not ask about it, nor was he offered the opportunity to learn about it. After his arrival, the parish nurse continued working with the youth without realizing what the youth pastor was thinking. One day the breaking point was reached and turf issues became very evident. He was thinking, "Why is this parish nurse invading my ministry?" while the parish nurse was thinking, "There is enough work for all of us. I love and am good at working with the youth concerning health and sexuality issues." Communication either had broken down or had never taken place. Once they were finally able to talk openly about their difficulties, they began to lead a youth group meeting together, tapping into each other's expertise and giftedness. This is just one example of the importance of communication, listening, and building trust. It is important to meet regularly to build and grow as a team.

Other areas of conflict may include a parishioner complaining to the parish nurse about the clergy, or vice versa; other staff undermining the parish health program; salary issues; and parishioners requesting one staff member to avoid contact with other staff (which will be addressed in the next section).

Inevitably, parishioners complain to one staff member about another. At such times, insecure staff members feel superior to other team members. It is important to remember that someone who complains about someone else will likely complain tomorrow to someone about us. These complaints should not be discounted, however, because they provide opportunities to listen to what the person is really saying. When deeper issues are explored, it can usually be traced to years of hurt within the church or the individual's own family. It is important not to be put in the middle; instead, offer to help the person practice techniques to face the one with whom he or she is angry. For support, you might offer to be present when the confrontation takes place. These can be times for growth and healing.

In addressing internal staff friction, we remember that evil is working strongly within and outside the church and the parish health program is not immune to it. Any growing program may be viewed as a threat by other staff. This is a time to listen and understand. Sometimes it is best, as some say, "to stay away from the water cooler."

Salary may be an area of conflict. In many churches, a low salary for clergy reflects the assumption that ministry is mission and that clergy should be willing to work for less. Nursing salaries have increased over the years and these may be considerably higher. If the nurse has been an employee of a hospital, it may be best for all parties if the nurse continues this employment contract, then the actual salary does not need to be disclosed (only the amount that the church contributes to the hospital for this ministry). In this situation the nurse's insurance, continuing education, and licensure remain the responsibility of the hospital and the church merely makes a contribution. Many times, the problem is not that the nurse is overpaid but that the clergy is underpaid.

Another issue of contention may be an on-call schedule. Pastors are expected to be on call twenty-four hours a day, seven days a week. In larger parishes, on-call duties are often shared among staff members. Is the nurse also on call twenty-four hours a day, seven days a week? In larger congregations, do nurses also take on-call shifts with clergy or do they just have office hours? These issues must be addressed at some point in the ongoing employment of the nurse.

WHEN TO PASS THE BALL

Important to any good juggling act is knowing when to pass the ball. Initially the clergy may see the parish nurse helping to carry his or her load in pastoral care, but within a matter of months, parishioners may be calling for the nurse rather than the clergy. If the nurse is dispensing spiritual care in addition to nursing care, where are those boundaries? Is it not the right of parishioners to ask for whomever they feel can provide what they need? At times the concern is in the realm of physical care, other times spiritual or emotional care. The parishioner, not the staff, always determines the initial need; yet sometimes the clergy or nurse may need to guide the parishioner to discover the real need.

A good working relationship means the responsibility bounces back and forth. For instance, either the nurse or the clergy could initially visit a parishioner in the hospital, possibly in relationship with the hospital chaplain, to discuss the parishioner's situation. After talking with the parishioner, the clergy may refer the situation to the parish nurse because hospice, extended rehabilitation, or a nursing home is needed. The nurse can assist with arrangements and details. Later, the nurse may identify deeper spiritual problems or realize that death is imminent and solicit clergy involvement. This cooperation utilizes the giftedness in each professional. A parish nurse can also be a great asset in involving the extended family of the parishioner, especially in the case of elderly parishioners. The parish nurse can be an excellent asset in working closely with the hospital. The relationships the nurse has established in that community can be invaluable to the care and understanding of the parishioner's needs. As this demonstrates, one of the most important concepts here is the team—the ability of the nurse and the pastor to share responsibilities and to support each other in the care of the parishioner and/or the parishioner's family.

ADDING MORE BALLS

Just as the juggler does not add more balls to his or her act until after having mastered the number currently being juggled, so with the parish health ministry. Add more program elements only when the existing ones are stable or completed. In adding programs, determine congregational needs and the extent of support. Add one program at a time without overextending.

EVALUATION

Constantly evaluate the program. Input from clients, participants, members of the congregation, and staff is essential. When evaluations are solicited, participants feel their opinions are valued, and they take ownership in the program. This results in the stabilization of human and financial resources for the health ministry. Evaluation can include personal stories, bulletin comment cards, letters from participants, or evaluation sheets at each parish health program or event. One church happens to have a donated massage table and a parishioner who is a massage therapist willing to donate a free monthly massage. Each month a drawing is held for a free massage and on the entry slip parishioners are asked to respond to the following: "Comments, ideas, suggestions about the Parish Health Program." This is a fun and easy way to get input from congregational members and discover some of their needs.

THE SHOW MUST GO ON

In this chapter we have addressed some programmatic parish health issues. We have suggested some ideas and actions in response to these issues and ways to promote the growth of parish health ministry. But we have not addressed one issue—the wind. Picture this. The jugglers (clergy and nurses) are standing on firm ground, with balls (parishioners and programs) circling through the air. But what about the wind? We picture this wind, not as a turbulent, unplanned gush of air that will make the balls fly in all directions, but rather as a gentle supportive wind, the Holy Spirit, offering guidance and direction. It is a wind that comes from prayer and placing our trust for the success of parish health ministry squarely in that spirit. Jesus reminded his disciples and daily reminds us that we are planters of seeds, but God is the one who provides the growth. Thanks be to God!

Chapter 10

Invitation to a Shared
Community Ministry

Judy Raley
Barbara Weinhold

Today's health care environment, with shorter hospital stays, more acutely ill patients, and an increasing emphasis on outpatient medicine, presents new challenges to spiritual caregivers. How do we assess and prioritize spiritual needs in this environment? How can our individual visions of ministry be expanded to complement one another? How can we collaborate as professionals and offer a continuum of spiritual care, in sickness and in health, to people of faith in our communities?

The changes in health care come at a time of increased interest in the relationship between spirituality and health. For example, a 1996 ICR Research Poll reveals that 736 out of the 1,000 interviewees believe that personal prayer or other spiritual and religious practices can speed healing and help the medical treatment of the ill. Thirty-four percent believe that prayer should be a standard part of the practice of medicine. A study at Duke University Medical Center (Koenig, Pargament, and Nielson, 1998) shows that seeking a connection with God staves off depression and improves life quality—despite the seriousness of the illness. In a 2000 Research Report, Dr. David Larson, psychiatrist and president of the National Institute for Healthcare Research, states, "The enhanced coping skills and better recoveries of the religious patient are some of the most overlooked, yet significant, factors in modern health care."

HEALTH CARE CHAPLAINS AND SPIRITUAL CARE

Health care chaplains focus on the spiritual dimension as integral to the healing process. They are pastoral care specialists with training and expertise to bring the presence and comfort of the divine to the health care environment. They serve as members of interdisciplinary teams and coordinators of spiritual care. Due to their training in spirituality and knowledge about health care systems, chaplains can identify patient needs and assist pastors in follow-up plans.

Illness brings people face-to-face with important issues. Chaplains help them assess their lives and focus their emotional and spiritual support. Chaplains are also trained to ascertain the patient's support system and how those relationships can assist the healing process.

Chaplains help patients identify and access resources to meet spiritual needs. They serve as a vital link between patients, community clergy, and other spiritual caregivers because they know the health care system and can assist clergy and family members with their questions and concerns, including help with setting up advance directives for health care. Chaplains serve as resources to churches to help volunteers with concerns about spirituality, aid team communication and referral skills, develop spiritual assessments, and visit people who are ill. Some chaplains are skilled in spiritual direction or in complementary therapies such as healing touch. They also facilitate support groups, such as those concerning grief, loss, and continuing support during chronic illness.

Today's health care environment calls for a paradigm shift for chaplains. Rather than simply identifying and responding to the spiritual needs of the hospitalized person, they must focus on wellness, prevention, education, early intervention, and care outside the health care institution. In this new paradigm, the role of the church in providing holistic care is heightened when chaplains become one of the care coordinators.

ROLE OF THE CHURCH

Churches by definition engage in health promotion because spiritual care is integral to health. Churches foster conditions in which people can grow and flourish as well as care for those who suffer illness and loss. They do this by encouraging people to pray, worship in song, reflect on questions of ultimate meaning, socialize, and commit themselves in service to the community. Faith has always been at the heart of health; belief and trust are central to healing. Saint John (10:10) quotes Jesus as saying, "I came that they might have life and have it to the full" (*The New American Bible,* 1970). Life is a gift from God and we are stewards of that gift.

The influence of Descartes's dualistic philosophy prevalent in the scientific community, however, tries to separate body and spirit. The church was to engage in the spiritual dimension of health while science and medicine dealt with the physical. In contrast, the church has long recognized the important connection between faith and health. Scriptural support for this holistic approach is found in James 5:14-16:

> Are any of you sick? Then call for the elders of the church, and have them pray over those who are sick and anoint them with oil in the name of Christ. And this prayer offered in faith will make them well, and Christ will raise them up. If they have sinned, they will be forgiven. So confess your sins to one another, and pray for one another, that you may be healed. The prayers of the just are powerful and effective (*The Inclusive New Testament,* 1994).

Recognizing that healing begins within the faith community, health care chaplains seek to establish networks with churches and synagogues to provide a community-based continuum of care.

PARISH NURSE MINISTRY

Parish nurse programs bring together churches and sponsoring health care facilities. In Parish Nurse Preparation Programs, nurses learn pastoral care skills and the importance of the faith-health connection in healing. The role of the parish nurse and the concept of team ministry of pastors and nurses are explained. This information enables pastors and nurses to work together, providing a continuity of pastoral care. In addition to providing a health ministry with screenings and health education, parish nurses can respond to spiritual needs. Most parishioners expect their pastor to be with them in a crisis situation and this is an important role of the clergy. Many ministers, however, are not able to continue regular visitation after the crisis has passed because of other demands on their time. The parish nurse is able to provide this follow-up support.

Local pastors and health care chaplains often serve as faculty for Parish Nurse Preparation Programs. In this way, the parish nurses become acquainted with spiritual leaders from both the health care setting and the community. These relationships encourage referrals to and by parish nurses of church members who can benefit from this continued spiritual support. In addition to the growing collaboration between nurses and clergy, physicians are increasingly suggesting care for the spiritual needs of their patients.

A 1998 survey by Daaleman and Frey revealed that 80 percent of U.S. family physicians refer their patients to clergy, with 30 percent making such referrals as often as ten or more times per year. A study the following year (Daaleman and Frey, 1999) found that 77 percent of hospital patients wanted doctors to consider their spiritual needs and nearly half, 48 percent, wanted their doctors to pray with them.

WEAVING A SHARED MINISTRY

The collaboration of health care chaplains, parish clergy, and parish nurses is a woven tapestry, a popular symbol in our time because people yearn to create wholeness out of fragmentation. A tapestry symbolizes the intertwining of our lives together, combining individual gifts to create a ministry stronger than any one of its strands.

Clergy Residency Programs

One way of enhancing the relationship between physicians and spiritual care providers in the setting served by these authors is through weeklong hospital residency programs for clergy. Hospital chaplains, physicians, and other staff join together to provide information to clergy that helps them provide support to their congregants who are affected by cancer and heart disease. Through several days of intensive lectures, facility tours, surgery observations, patient visitations, and group discussions, participants gain a better understanding of how cancer and heart disease impact the total person. The chaplains lead discussions on spirituality, communication skills, assessment, and referral skills. The parish nurse coordinator talks with the clergy participants about the parish nurse program. These residencies acknowledge the roles of community clergy and parish nurses as integral to the healing team and acquaint them with resources available to them in the health care system.

The response has been enthusiastic. "This was one of the most dynamic, most mind-stretching experiences I have ever encountered," one clergy related. "I can now explain some of the terminology and better ease the anxiety of my parishioners. I can assure them of the excellence of the care provided by the physicians and the hospital."

A health care system chaplain relates how collaboration and the clergy residency experience helped a clergy with a crisis situation in which a parishioner in the surgical intensive care unit became critically ill and the chaplain called the family clergy:

> When the clergy arrived, I recognized him from previous visits he had made to other members of his church. He had also attended the cardiac residency program, which helps clergy better understand heart health and disease in order to minister more meaningfully to their church members with cardiac problems. I briefed the clergy on what was happening as we went into the intensive care unit. The entire family and two close friends were gathered around the patient's bed. I lingered in the background as the pastor greeted all the family. Then he took the hand of the patient and asked everyone to join hands as he bowed his head in prayer. He waved to me to come closer, and the family members reached out their hands for me to join them. After prayer, as the family was talking about their loved one, many tears were shed. The clergy told us a touching story about the patient, and I knew with certainty that he knew his flock. Before I slipped out, I told the family that the staff could contact me for further help, and I let the nurse know that the minister had arrived and was with the family. The nurse contacted me when the patient expired, and I immediately went to the family and the clergy to offer my assistance. I answered their questions about what would happen next, including the doctor's pronouncement of death, the release papers to be signed, and the necessary contact with the funeral home. I showed them a quiet room where they could gather and

a phone they could use if they needed to contact anyone. A few weeks later when I saw this clergy, I told him how privileged I was to minister with him and his church family. He told me that he was just becoming comfortable in the hospital setting. He appreciated how welcoming and comforting the staff had been, and he was especially grateful for the cardiac residency, which helped him to see hospitals and its care in a whole new way.

Another Collaboration in Practice

The following scenario offers a glimpse of the tapestry woven by a hospital chaplain, a clergy, and parish nurse as they worked together to provide a continuum of spiritual care:

Jim found both peace and help through a network of spiritual caregivers in his church and the hospital when he was admitted with a serious heart condition. Following a cardiology consultation to determine his status as a heart transplant candidate, he was released to home care. The next month he returned to the hospital in critical condition. During the chaplain's visit, Jim revealed that both parents and a sibling had died at an early age and he felt that he too would die young. He had been reflecting on his spiritual life and was concerned. Several years prior to this hospitalization he had started the Rite of Christian Initiation of Adults (RCIA) class with the intent of being baptized in the Catholic Church. Ill health prevented him from continuing the RCIA process at that time, but now he wished to complete the classes and be baptized. Sensing the importance and urgency of this request, the chaplain called the priest at the parish where Jim had begun the RCIA process. The priest visited and Jim was able to receive Baptism, Confirmation, Eucharist, and the Sacrament of the Anointing of the Sick. As this cherished dream came true, he exhibited a sense of deep peace. Receiving daily Communion was the highlight of his day and he always had his rosary with him in the hospital. The chaplain visited regularly with Jim during his hospital stay. A referral was also given to the parish nurse at Jim's church. The parish nurse continued to provide spiritual support for Jim when he was dismissed to hospice care at home and later entered a nursing home.

DOES IT ALWAYS WORK?

This all sounds good, but does it always work? Of course, it does not. There are many barriers to this kind of shared ministry. Unclear lines of communication can inhibit the exchange of information needed for continual spiritual care. Health care chaplains need to know who the parish nurses are and how to contact them. Parish nurses and local clergy need to know the chaplains and their service areas. When ministers or parish nurses are unable to get to the hospital, they need to be able to call the chaplains directly and request that their parishioners be visited. This lets the patients know that the ministers are concerned and that they are not forgotten or ignored.

The education of congregational members about spiritual resources available to them is also an important ingredient in collaboration. In turn, the pastor or church secretary must notify the parish nurse of congregational needs. If chaplains are not aware of patient situations, either through a direct request or from their pastor, they may not visit. If the chaplain does not call the pastor when a patient with spiritual needs is discharged, the continuity of care for those needs may be broken.

Lack of trust can be a barrier to this vision of shared community ministry. Relationship-building activities for community clergy, chaplains, and parish nurses are important in establishing a mutual level of confidence for each professional group. Chaplaincy departments can invite local clergy to breakfasts to meet these spiritual caregivers and tell them about hospital services. Chaplains might serve as faculty for the community clinical pastoral education program. Hospital-sponsored community forums on topics such as Alzheimer's in the faith community, spirituality of aging, bioethics, managed care, and end-of-life issues bring together chaplains, parish nurses, clergy, and physicians. Each encounter can build trust and increase the potential for continual spiritual support, from home to hospital and back to home, for members of our community.

Other factors may hinder the development of community ministry. Some individuals committed to spiritual care and holistic health work better alone. They are uncomfortable, and probably not effective, in this model of shared ministry. Some clergy do not understand that parish nurses and chaplains enhance, rather than dilute, the spiritual support and growth available to their members. Chaplains need to begin to think of ministry beyond the health care facility and see patients as members of a congregation and community who are temporarily in their care.

ACHIEVING A CONTINUUM OF SPIRITUAL CARE

Collaboration is key to this shared ministry. All those involved need to examine their own gifts and skills to see where they best fit and what they can offer. The Myers-Briggs Type Indicator is a useful tool for both personal and team development. Building a team of professionals who trust one another is vital to the success of any collaborative effort.

We are all beginners in this vision of shared community ministry, but we are inspired by the thoughts of Thomas Merton (1971) about beginners: "We do not want to be beginners. But let us be convinced of the fact that we will never be anything else but beginners all our lives" (p. 37).

REFERENCES

Daaleman, Timothy P. and Frey, Bruce (1998). Prevalence and patterns of physician referral to clergy and pastoral care providers. *Archives of Family Medicine, 7*, 548-553.

Daaleman, Timothy P. and Frey, Bruce (1999). Spiritual and religious beliefs and practices of family physicians: A national survey. *The Journal of Family Practice, 48*(2), 98-104.

Health Enhanced by Faith. National Institute of Healthcare Research (2000). Research Report, <http://www.nihr.org/researchreports/healthfaith.html>.

ICR Research Group (1996). Faith and health poll. *USA Weekend,* February 16-20.

The Inclusive New Testament (1994). Hyattsville, MD: Priests for Equality.

Koenig, Harold G., Pargament, Kenneth L., and Nielson, Julie (1998). Religious coping and health status in medically ill hospitalized older adults. *Journal of Nervous and Mental Disease, 186*(9), 513-521.

Merton, Thomas (1971). *Contemplative Prayer.* Garden City, NY: Doubleday, p. 37.

The New American Bible (1970). Washington DC: Confraternity of Christian Doctrine.

Chapter 11

Spiritual Care: Bridging the Disciplines in Congregational Health Ministries

Karen Hahn
James M. Radde
John E. Fellers

How do community clergy, health care chaplains, and congregational nurses collaborate within a health ministry when their roles overlap? These three professionals can collaborate, compete, or operate in parallel tracks.

This chapter uses spiritual care case studies to illustrate principles of collaboration and role definition in health ministry. It also describes key issues affecting role boundaries, functions, communication mechanisms, and understandings involved in providing effective spiritual care. Case presentations illustrate examples of collaborations and role violations. These cases clarify critical components of the role definitions and principles of effective collaboration.

TERMINOLOGY

The terms "parish nurse" and "congregational nurse" are used interchangeably to reflect regional and denominational preferences. The term "clergy" refers to ordained persons who serve in a congregational setting. The term "chaplain" refers to certified clergy or laypersons who serve in institutional health care settings.

Each of these professionals provides spiritual care. This is described as "a style and quality of presence to the sick person. Establishing a climate of acceptance and trust can, in the Lord's own time, help facilitate the interior revelation to the patient of what he or she needs right now" (Radde, 1984, pp. 15-16).

Role Descriptions

Overlapping roles call for clear description and differentiation. Parish nurses, chaplains, and community clergy all provide spiritual care to congregants. Descriptions of their roles and functions follow, and a series of hospital visitation case studies illustrates other factors that influence their roles.

How are professional roles described? They are described professionally, legally, relationally, and theologically. For example, parish nurses (Health Ministries Association and American Nurses Association, 1998) and chaplains (National Association of Catholic Chaplains [NACC], 1998) have published standards of practice developed by their respective professional organizations. Laws impact the practice of each profession, and the roles of each are further defined by institutional job descriptions. The judicatory bodies and doctrines of most denominations define the professional roles of clergy. Last, each of these roles is also determined by the gifts of individuals and how they relate to themselves, to God, to nature, and to other persons.

Professional Definitions

According to the International Parish Nurse Resource Center:

> Parish nursing is an emerging area of specialized professional nursing practice distinguished by the following characteristics: Parish nursing practice holds the spiritual dimension to be central to the practice. It also encompasses the physical, psychological, and social dimensions of nursing practice.
>
> The parish nurse role balances knowledge with skill; the sciences with theology and with the humanities; service with worship, and nursing care functions with pastoral care functions. . . . The focus of [parish nursing practice] is the faith community and its ministry. The parish nurse, in collaboration with the pastoral staff and congregational members, participates in the ongoing transformation of the faith community into a source of health and healing. Through partnership with other community

health resources, parish nursing fosters new and creative responses to health concerns. (Solari-Twadell, 1999, p. 15)

The late Lutheran minister Granger Westberg is the pioneer of chaplain training in the Texas Gulf Coast Region and father of the parish nurse movement. He describes (1999) the role functions of the parish nurse as "health educator . . . personal health counselor . . . referral agent . . . coordinator of volunteers . . . developer of support groups . . . [who] assists people to integrate faith and health, [and] . . . health advocate" (p. 38).

The NACC describes a chaplain as a board-certified professional who integrates spiritual care in the promotion of health and wellness. Chaplain role functions include facilitating theological reflection in persons of faith groups other than the chaplain's; helping others discover meaning in their suffering; assisting others in applying their own values in decision making; communicating with other disciplines; collaborating on an interdisciplinary team; and facilitating complementary healing modalities. The Joint Commission on Accreditation of Hospital Organizations (JCAHO) is negotiating with the Association of Professional Chaplains (APC) and NACC to set a standard for the term "certified chaplain."

The role of clergy in a parish or congregational setting usually focuses on three areas: proclaimer, priestly figure, and pastor. The proclaimer/prophetic role is most often expressed through preaching and teaching insights from scripture and religious tradition. The priestly role contains sacramental celebrations, such as communion and baptism. This role is also expressed in leading liturgies and presiding at life events such as marriage and burial. At its most basic level, the priestly role is one that stands at the intersection of the divine-human encounter to help the faith community relive its faith story.

The pastoral function of clergy is, in some sense, the most complex of the three. It involves interaction with persons particularly in times of crisis such as illness, death, relational breakups, and personal traumas. It also embraces a more pedestrian expression by simply projecting the presence of an entire religious community into everyday events and social encounters through a designated representative. J. F. Hopewell (1990) gives an excellent summary of the clergy's work in the *Dictionary of Pastoral Care and Counseling*. He wrote, "Whether by ritual, hospitality, consolation, or advice, the pastor tries to make matters whole: to give integrity to lives, solidarity to groups, to mend broken relationships, to heal, accept, [and] restore" (p. 827).

Legal Boundaries

Legal boundaries help define the respective roles of these professionals. For example, the specialty practice of parish nursing is delimited by the Nurse Practice Act of each state as well as by the American Nurses Association. Institutional job descriptions further define specific professional roles.

Laws require the reporting of suspected child abuse. These laws affect nurses, chaplains, and community clergy. States also have laws related to confidentiality. In Oregon, Father Mockaitis, a Roman Catholic priest, and his bishop, Archbishop George, filed suit against the district attorney and others for taping a prisoner participating in the Sacrament of Reconciliation (i.e., during confession). The judge remanded to the district court an injunction that prohibited any recording of "confidential communication from inmates of the county jail to any member of the clergy in the member's professional character" (*Mockaitis v. Harcleroad,* 1997). The Baz case, which will be described later, helped clarify the chaplain's role by ruling that proselytizing was not an appropriate role function (*Baz v. Walters,* 1986).

Relational Role Definitions

Relational as well as legal factors affect role descriptions. When functions overlap in spiritual care, such as in the area of counseling, the role definitions must be determined relationally. In some evangelical traditions, the role of the clergy and other church leaders is determined relationally—in response to the call of a particular faith community.

Other relational components affecting role descriptions include other pastoral team roles, caseload, individual gifts, educational preparation, areas of authority, personal preferences, and client preferences. In one congregation, the clergy may expect the parish nurse to provide leadership in health visitation and pastoral counseling. That nurse might need to obtain additional training in pastoral counseling. In another congregation, the care team coordinator might oversee health visitation and a licensed counselor provide the pastoral counseling, thus freeing the nurse for other health ministry functions such as health counselor.

Theological Definitions

Finally, theology and tradition often determine role functions. For example, in certain denominations the ministerial roles of women and men are clearly differentiated. Some faith traditions distinguish between the roles and functions of ordained and unordained, especially in their sacramental and liturgical aspects. Under certain conditions, church doctrine may allow laypersons to distribute communion. The various certifying bodies determine the theological dimensions of a chaplain's role.

MINISTRY EVENTS

The following case studies describe actual ministry events that highlight principles related to role definition and collaboration. Details are changed to protect confidentiality.

Collaboration Case Study: Patrick

Patrick's neck was broken two months ago as he changed a flat tire by the side of the highway; he has been on a rehabilitation unit of a large hospital in an urban medical center for almost three weeks. He has been told that he will be quadriplegic for the rest of his life, unable to walk or totally care for himself. He flies into rages with staff members, hurling obscenities and food trays across the ward. No family member has visited or called.

Patrick is a new member of a small evangelical congregation which teaches that if he believes, he will be healed. Staff members try to encourage him to "be realistic" and "learn to live with his limitations," but he refuses to work with them. He cooperates with only one occupational therapist, one physical therapist, and one nurse on the day and evening shifts. He says he likes them because they "pray with me for healing; I'm going to get better." When these staff persons are off duty, he sulks or throws tantrums.

The nursing staff went to the chaplain for help. Chaplain Bob began visiting him daily, and Patrick tolerates his visits since the chaplain carefully chose to pray in ways that support hope and strengthen his faith but do not contradict his beliefs in faith healing. Staff members welcome the chaplain's visits.

Patrick's clergy visits once a week and prays with him for faith healing, reinforcing Patrick's attempts to expect full physical healing. He also provides instruction on the week's lessons and Bible readings. Staff members tend to avoid Patrick after these visits because he becomes belligerent and easily defensive.

At the request of Patrick's clergy, the congregational nurse from the coalition of churches visits him once a week. Carol believes that miracles do happen but that they happen rarely. She does not believe that sufficient faith produces healing. Carol brings Patrick the church newsletter, the tape of the service, the Bible readings, and teachings for the week. She prays with Patrick for healing but does not specify physical healing.

Although initially hesitant, nursing staff members accept Carol because she makes special efforts to empathize with them and helps them understand Patrick's perspective. Nurses comment that Patrick is more "cooperative" after her visits.

They have asked Carol to speak with the clergy about "not reinforcing his negative attitude." They lack rapport with Patrick and hope that Carol can help. Carol consents, hoping to facilitate healing on the nursing unit and to promote a more therapeutic environment for Patrick.

Ideally, Carol could have facilitated a collaborative team approach by requesting a staffing that included the clergy, the nursing staff, and the chaplain. Instead, she consults with Chaplain Bob in an effort to understand better the dynamics between the clergy and nursing staff members.

Carol already has an appointment scheduled with Chaplain Bob to ask whether he believes the book *A Step Further* might be helpful to Patrick (Eareckson and Estes, 1978). Co-authored by a quadriplegic who was not healed from her physical paralysis, the author travels all over the world giving her testimony and demonstrating her mouthbrush artwork.

The chaplain approves the book as a therapeutic tool after discussing it with the clergy. Staff members provide Patrick with a mouthstick with which to turn the book pages. This book becomes the critical link between the staff and Patrick as he reads portions of it aloud to them. They learn to dialogue with Patrick about the book with the help of Chaplain Bob.

The therapists, the day nurse, and the evening nurse whom Patrick likes have modeled their praying with Patrick on the chaplain's ecumenical perspective. None of them believe in faith healing. However, they all have found ways of praying with Patrick that are mutually satisfying. Patrick likes them because he feels supported in his spiritual as well as his emotional and physical healing.

Discussion of the Case

What has happened here? The chaplain has modeled ways of praying and supporting hope with Patrick that are acceptable to all of the staff. The chaplain has also provided a daily dose of predictable spiritual and emotional support for Patrick, support which both the staff and Patrick rely on to improve their adaptations. Staff members have also found support in the chaplain's nonjudgmental listening to their frustrations and in his quieting presence for them and for Patrick.

The nursing staff members have found someone they hope will mediate their differences and discomfort with the clergy and his theological stance—the congregational nurse—just as the chaplain helped to mediate their differences with the patient. The nurse links the patient in his present situation to the patient as person in his everyday life, to his faith community, and to the nursing staff. The parish nurse has advocated for Patrick with the nursing staff and has facilitated communication and understanding among the different team members.

The clergy has faithfully fulfilled his role as shepherd and teacher, instructing his new member in the teachings of his church. His hospital visits have been vital to strengthening Patrick's new relationship with a church that he had joined because he liked the theological perspective, the way of praying, and the support.

Ultimately there was a happy ending. Patrick did walk out of the hospital—on full leg braces. Patrick learned to tolerate and even work with almost all members of the staff. The clergy continued to support Patrick's new faith and added additional partners to Patrick's healing team—the church music ministers. The parish nurse elicited the cooperation of the hospital staff in allowing the music ministry team to play and sing for the entire unit. This became a weekly event that all enjoyed.

This case study highlights two aspects of professional and relational roles:

1. Provide spiritual care within the context of professional definitions of scope and standards of practice.
2. Define team member roles in relation to such aspects as the setting of the encounter, the nature of each team member's relationship to the patient, and the unique gifts of each team member.

Collaboration Case Study: William

William calls his community clergy to say that he is having an angiogram in the morning. He attends Mass daily and knows the priest well. He wants the priest to visit him before his procedure. Father Bill, the priest, has commitments he cannot break, but he contacts the parish nurse. Maria, the volunteer Catholic parish nurse, cannot visit William either. She calls the hospital's pastoral care department, leaving a general request for a chaplain to visit because she does not know any of the chaplains personally. A chaplain fills this request, visiting him before the procedure.

Following the procedure, William is hospitalized for three weeks because of heart surgery and complications. Maria visits him after surgery and encourages him to request daily Communion if he wants it. Father Bill, not able to visit because he is pastoring a congregation of over 2,000 members, phones William to give him support. A Roman Catholic lay minister comes every day from one of the area churches and brings him the Eucharist.

William makes friends with all of the nurses. He jokes about chasing them in his sneakers as he does his prescribed walking exercises around the nurses' station. He returns home from the hospital with a list of medications and five bottles of pills. Maria visits him in his home just as she visits high-risk patients after discharge. She finds out that William cannot drive yet and cannot figure out a system for taking his medications. At discharge the staff saw no need for a home health nurse referral.

The parish nurse sets up a medication management system for William. She helps him sort out what behavior changes are needed for him to lead a more healthy lifestyle. He believes that God "just needed to hit me over the head with a two-by-four to get my attention, and this heart surgery is my two-by-four." William asks Maria to bring Communion when she visits him because he believes the sacrament will help him to heal. She asks her priest to authorize her to be a lay minister of Communion. Maria brings William Communion until he is able to drive himself to daily Mass again.

Discussion of the Case

This case study highlights how theological stances can also affect role definition. The priest has provided pastoral leadership by inviting the parish nurse to respond to William's pastoral needs. The parish nurse has provided spiritual care by helping William integrate his faith and health concerns. In addition to these, she has provided services within her role functions of health counselor and educator. The hospital chaplain has provided the presence and prayer requested by the patient. The surrounding parishes, through their coordinated scheduling of Communion, have helped meet William's sacramental needs.

PRINCIPLES OF EFFECTIVE COLLABORATION

These two case studies illustrate the following principles of effective collaboration:

- Acknowledge and maximize the use of one another's gifts.
- Respect and accept one another's theological and other differences.

- Include one another in developing and implementing the plan of care when indicated.
- Respect geographical areas of responsibility and authority.
- Mutually determine role boundaries when overlap occurs.
- Coordinate the plan of care around demonstrated needs so that it supports the client, providing hope, growth, and healing in multiple dimensions.
- Honor confidentiality while communicating about the client's needs and responses.

ROLE VIOLATIONS

Role boundaries can be further defined by describing inappropriate behaviors.

Parish Nurse Role Violation Case Study

Harriet, a patient in a long-term acute care facility for forty-three days, is recovering from an amputation followed by multiple life-threatening complications. She has just been weaned from a ventilator and is learning to talk again. She told the parish nurse, also a member of her church, that she is very angry with God. She said that she does not want anyone to pray for her because she does not believe in God anymore and does not "believe in prayer." She does not want to "talk to a God who would do this to me."

Furthermore, Harriet does not want her clergy to visit because she has also "quit the church." She accepts the visits of the congregational nurse, Kathy, because she is teaching her communication techniques and "does not talk about God or faith." Instead, the nurse prays silently and provides a pastoral presence during her weekly visits.

Kathy continues to communicate with the clergy about Harriet's overall condition and spiritual response because she wishes his support in reaching out to Harriet. Also, she is hopeful that Harriet's rejection of church affiliation is a temporary response to her illness.

The parish nurse is trained to provide spiritual care that is compatible with the religious beliefs of individuals. This includes honoring their choice not to belong to a church and to exclude a clergy from their care. Kathy violated client confidentiality by consulting with the pastor after Harriet had clearly stated she was no longer a church member. She might have avoided this problem if she had asked Harriet's permission to communicate with her clergy.

Chaplain Role Violation Case Study

An ordained minister, Franklin Baz (*Baz v. Walters,* 1986) was hired as a chaplain at the Veterans Administration Medical Center in Danville, Illinois, in

1977. Baz turned a Sunday evening musical recreation period for patients into a Christian evangelical service at which he preached and proselytized. At times he interfered with decisions made by the medical staff. On several occasions he entered the surgical amphitheater without permission in order to pray for patients.

Reverend Baz's employment was terminated in less than a year because he failed to collaborate. Baz sued for reinstatement and back pay. He claimed his rights had been violated because he was required by his religious affiliation, the Assemblies of God, to live out specific theological beliefs and practices, namely, preaching and proselytizing. The Veterans Administration prohibits proselytizing and any imposition of ministry. Baz lost his case in district court and his appeals as well.

Pastor Role Violation Case Study

A local clergy entered the hospital room of a ten-year-old boy recovering from burns who was not a member of his congregation. He pointed his finger at the boy and said, "It's your sins that have caused this!" A nurse reported the incident to the chaplain who alerted hospital security officers. They traced the car license number and provided the clergy's name to the chaplain. The chaplain phoned him to set up an appointment, but he refused to meet with the chaplain. The chaplain, security guard, and nursing staff met and planned how they would prevent any future intrusions if he should return. The clergy overstepped his boundaries by imposing a moral judgment on the boy, a patient who was not a member of his congregation.

CONCLUSION

All three members of a health ministry team—clergy, chaplains, and congregational nurses—collaborate in providing pastoral care and counseling, assuming they have the requisite skills and training. Clear role descriptions are vital. How will they determine who will provide what services? This will depend upon the setting, which of them is available, which of them has the necessary training, and the personal gifts of the providers. No matter how they decide to proceed, their decision must be acceptable to the client.

Role functions unique to one member of the pastoral care team, such as certain sacramental functions, are not difficult to identify and differentiate. In such cases, team members must know when to refer. They may also need to coordinate the pastoral activities within the routine of the hospital. Familiarity with, and sensitivity to, the various religious traditions is essential.

Examining role violations helps to clarify role descriptions and appropriate role boundaries. It is the responsibility of health care and pastoral team members to protect the well-being of clients regardless of setting.

Effective collaboration requires following some simple rules:

- Place God and the client first.
- Respect one another's gifts.
- Respond to the client's preferences and needs.
- Communicate with one another.
- Reserve territoriality for the endangered species.
- Respect one another's differences.
- Communicate about mutual expectations and about areas of potential overlap.
- Plan together.
- Periodically evaluate the effectiveness of working relationships.

Effective collaboration introduces unique challenges, but the time and commitment reap benefits for the professionals as well as the clients. Collaboration offers a hopeful antidote to the depersonalization that pervades so much of the contemporary health care industry.

REFERENCES

Baz v. Walters (1986). 782 F.2d 701 (7th Cir.).

Eareckson, J. and Estes, S. (1978). *A step further.* Grand Rapids, MI: Zondervan Publishing House.

Health Ministries Association and American Nurses Association (1998). *Scope and standards of parish nursing practice.* Washington, DC: American Nurses Publishing.

Hopewell, J. F. (1990). Pastor. In Hunter, R. J. (Ed.), *Dictionary of pastoral care and counseling* (p. 827). Nashville, TN: Abingdon Press.

Mockaitis v. Harcleroad (1997). 104 F. 3rd 1522 (9th Cir.).

National Association of Catholic Chaplains (1998). *Standards.* May. Milwaukee, WI. #400-420.5.

Radde, J. M. (1984). Preparing to give spiritual care. *Journal of Christian Healing, 6,* 15-16.

Solari-Twadell, P. A. (1999). The emerging practice of parish nursing. In Solari-Twadell, P. A. and McDermott, M. A. (Eds.), *Parish nursing—Promoting whole person health within faith communities* (p. 15). London: Sage Publications.

Westberg, G. (1999). A personal historical perspective of whole person health and the congregation. In Solari-Twadell, P. A. and McDermott, M.A. (Eds.), *Parish nursing—Promoting whole person health within faith communities* (p. 38). London: Sage Publications.

Chapter 12

Faith Community Nursing and Health Care Chaplaincy in Australia: A New Collaboration

Anne Van Loon
Lindsay B. Carey

Across Australia numerous health care chaplains, parish clergy, and nurses of religious faith have willingly collaborated for many years. This collaboration has sought to ensure a continuity of appropriate physical, spiritual, and emotional care, not only for people within health care settings, but also for those requiring additional support in their local community.

In general, however, the success of such collaboration has varied enormously, depending upon the epistemological ethos of health care organizations and the philosophical-religious viewpoints of policy decision makers on church councils and among government authorities at local, state, and/or national levels. Inadequate cooperation among these various factions has, more often than not, resulted either in nonexistent or substandard spiritual, emotional, and physical care for the majority of patients and their families. This is particularly true for those in the community who fall into the gaps between caregiving organizations.

Thus, the development of faith community nursing (FCN) in Australia is timely. It can provide the badly needed specialized ministry of combined physical and spiritual care by creatively linking health care chaplains, parish clergy, and the nursing profession with those in the community needing support.

FAITH COMMUNITY NURSING IN AUSTRALIA

While nurses have worked in specific faith communities in Australia for many years, their increased involvement in pastoral care and health ministry in a more structured way commenced as recently as 1996. At that time, a public seminar attended by 100 people introduced the concept of FCN to church and nursing professionals in South Australia. All seminar participants were invited to join in a demonstration project to develop a model of FCN that was tailored to Australia's social, cultural, and religious context. While the invitation to join the project went to many faith communities, only Christian groups responded (Van Loon, 1999).

The FCN pilot project commenced in February 1997 in Adelaide, the capital city of South Australia, using four South Australian congregations (one Anglican, two Roman Catholic, one Lutheran) working with one ecumenical faith community agency that helped homeless youth. Two parishes were located in metropolitan Adelaide and two in a semirural township, varying in size from fewer than 100 to 3,000 members. All the faith community nurses (FCNs) volunteered up to twelve hours per week. The congregations received small local government grants ($A1000-3,000) to cover start-up expenses, but the faith communities bear most of the continuation expenses.

One present author and twelve additional professionals, including nurses, doctors, parish clergy, and chaplains, established and incorporated the Australian Faith Community Nurses Association (AFCNA) at the same time as the demonstration project began. Its mandate was to provide the following:

- FCN promotion and publicity
- Continuing education focusing on spirituality and health issues
- Peer support
- Resource development and distribution
- Consultancy
- Political action, including lobbying

The AFCNA, during 1997, 1998, and 2000, developed and conducted, in conjunction with Luther Seminary (Adelaide, South Australia), a one-week course titled "Introduction to Faith Community Nursing" to prepare registered nurses for a ministry of health, healing, and wholeness within a local faith community. This course used guidelines developed by the International Parish Nurse Resource Center (United States) to ensure an international best practice standard for faith community nursing in Australia (Table 12.1).

TABLE 12.1. Content of Australian Faith Community Nurse Training Course

The Faith Community Nurse Role	Functions of the FCN
I. History of faith community nursing	I. Education
II. Scope and models of FCN	II. Counseling
III. Philosophy of the FCN role	III. Resource and Referral
	IV. Advocacy
	V. Care Coordination
Spiritual Contexts of Practice	**Accountability and Confidentiality**
I. Care as vocation	I. Documentation and information systems
II. Spiritual formation	II. Legal, liability, and ethical issues
	III. Evaluation techniques (self/program)
	IV. Professional standards of practice
Ministering to the Faith Community	**Practice Management Issues**
I. Integration of faith and health	I. Working with volunteers
II. God and suffering	II. Time limits
III. Pastoral care	III. Budgets and conducting meetings
Assessing Your Faith Community	**Health Promotion and Illness Prevention**
I. Physical and spiritual needs assessment	I. Process, resources, and referral
II. Faith community as client	II. Developing programs
III. Ethics and responsible care	III. Special needs groups and crisis intervention
Developing Community Transformation	**Spiritual Leadership and and Personal Care**
I. Values clarification	I. Self-care
II. Community empowerment	II. Prayer
III. Working ecumenically	III. Worship

SOCIAL AND RELIGIOUS CONTEXT IN AUSTRALIA

During the process of establishing the AFCNA, it became apparent that major differences in the structures of Australian and U.S. health systems, plus social, cultural, and religious differences, necessitated an adaptation of the parish nurse model originating from North America (Westberg, 1989, 1990; Westberg and Westberg McNamara, 1990). Australia has a population of approximately 18 million people (Australian Bureau of Statistics, 1996). Kaldor et al. (1999, pp. 7-9) noted that although two-thirds of Australians consider religion and spirituality "important" and nearly three-quarters "believe in God" (74 percent), only one-fifth (20 percent) attend a faith community more than once per month. Active members of non-Christian religions such as Buddhism, Judaism, and Islam comprise only 2.66 percent of the population; those with "no religion" or not stating a religion, 25.6 percent. This latter number increased by 35 percent between the 1991 and 1996 census (Hughes et al., 1995). The Australian National Church Life Survey (NCLS) (Kaldor et al., 1994, 1997) notes that traditional denominational allegiance and attendance continue to decline.

These results suggest three trends pertinent to the development of FCN in Australia. The Anglican, Roman Catholic, and Uniting Church denominations (which together make up over half the Christian population) experience less regular church attendance and active participation, especially in the under-forty-year-old age group. People under forty look for churches that meet their relevant needs. The National Church Life Survey (NCLS) (Kaldor et al., 1997, pp. 186-195) indicates that the two most valued aspects of congregational life are "spiritual nurture" and "caring." Newcomers to the church highly value the feeling of being "part of a *caring* congregation." Parishes with established FCNs have the tremendous advantage of ensuring ongoing care to young adults and their families when they require additional and special nurturing.

A second notable trend encouraging the development of FCN is the decline in numbers at religious services as a result of Australia's aging population. Currently 2.2 million Australians are over the age of sixty-five years and this number will rise to 5.5 million by 2041 (Hughes, 1999). This substantial number of retired persons, many of whom are being cared for at home or within elder care facilities, means that regular contact with local parishes will greatly diminish.

FCNs can ensure regular ongoing physical and spiritual support for these older people.

The Australian Chaplaincy Utility Research project (Carey, 1995; Carey, Aroni, and Edwards, 1997) undertaken at the Royal Children's Hospital in Melbourne suggested the need for a third factor in collaboration. While the majority (88.2 percent) of participating doctors, nurses, and allied health staff appreciated chaplains as part of the hospital system, some noted the lack of pastoral care follow-up for the increasing number of patients who, for reasons of hospital economic efficiency, were being discharged early. Nearly one-third of the staff (32.1 percent) who believed that hospital chaplaincy services should continue reported that the chaplain's pastoral care role "could be extended" to include regular pastoral visits to the homes of discharged patients. They were particularly concerned for those who needed assistance in addressing personal or spiritual issues that challenged or disturbed them during their hospitalization. Given the increasing numbers of rapid patient discharges, most health care chaplains could not assume this responsibility, although this extension of pastoral care could be feasible with the help of FCNs and parish clergy.

Overall, these trends suggest that Australian churches need to develop a meaningful focus on the needs of their members and the wider community. Such new forms of ministry are fundamental to the churches' pastoral care, the dynamic growth of congregational life, and reaching the community. FCN is one definitive response.

In addition, FCN, as it seeks to reach the public and provide pastoral support within the Australian context, can potentially develop an "interministry" across and within numerous spheres of administration (Figure 12.1). This interministry between and within various organizations and associations can reduce bureaucratic red tape or administrative oversight and expedite the necessary primary care needed by patients and their families.

FCN has already identified three significant areas of collaboration although it is in its infancy. The first collaboration concerns supportive relationships between clergy, nurses, and health committees. The second is the importance of ongoing trust, support, and nurture among pastoral leaders that promotes open and authentic communication. The third collaborative area promotes a continuum of spiritual care by health care chaplains, hospital-based health professionals, and the congregational spiritual support team of the parish clergy and the

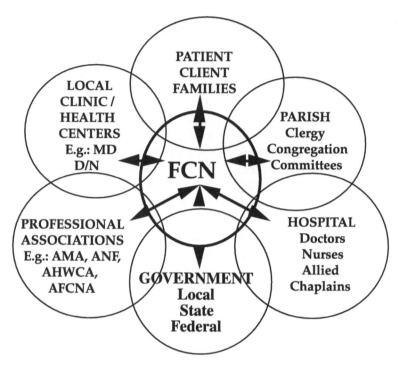

(MD = Medical Doctor; D/N = District Nurse; AMA = Australian Medical Association; AHWCA = Australian Health and Welfare Chaplains Association; ANA = Australian Nurses Federation; AFCNA = Australian Faith Community Nurses Association).

FIGURE 12.1. The "Interministry" of the Faith Community Nurse (FCN)

faith community nurses. A brief description of each collaborative area follows.

SUPPORTIVE RELATIONSHIPS AMONG CLERGY, NURSES, AND HEALTH COMMITTEES

Enthusiastic, supportive relationships were necessary to initiate faith community nursing (Van Loon, 1999). Several potential FCN centers were desperate to commence this ministry and join the demonstration project, but they found that the parish clergy did not share the FCN vision. These nurses were consequently unable to commence their work. Two of the nurses worked for twelve months with a local health committee supporting their efforts, only to be stymied by parish clergy.

Other faith communities were unable to gain momentum because parish clergy were ambivalent about FCN. They were not opposed, but hesitant about its role, functions, benefits, and financial sustainability. Nurses who received little encouragement and support from parish clergy often gave up. Most seemed willing to try for about twelve months, but if parish clergy and local leadership attitudes did not become more supportive, they ceased efforts. Conversely, many parish clergy and congregations were very keen and supportive, but FCNs were hesitant and unsure about their role. In such situations FCN never progressed beyond initial discussion stages. Such lack of support between pastors and nurses "flys in the face" of collaborations so earnestly encouraged for over forty years since the publication of Granger's *Nurse, Pastor, and Patient* (1955).

Successful FCN endeavors have highlighted important key issues. These include the need to articulate the benefits of the FCN health ministry for the members of the faith community, the parish clergy, and other local leaders. In this context, AFCNA, in conjunction with Sydney Adventist Hospital, produced a sixteen-minute promotional video (AFCNA, 1999a) that contains edited interviews with four nurses, parish clergy, the AFCNA president, and one client. Hopefully it will facilitate dialogue between leaders, nurses, and faith communities.

The AFCNA (1999b) produced a manual containing information required to facilitate initiation of an FCN program. Its purpose was to ensure appropriate professional FCN standards and to provide accurate information that would facilitate open discussion and decision making about proceeding with an FCN ministry. The manual includes documentation masters and information on all the requisite process issues.

The AFCNA considered it imperative that the roles and functions of the FCNs be clearly delineated from the outset. This clarity encouraged parish clergy to address how this role intersected with their own, how it matched the overall mission of the congregation, and how areas of responsibility were defined. Experience taught that tensions rose when FCNs became overloaded with difficult pastoral care cases. While some members of the congregation or community will strain the available human resources excessively, this is less a problem when the burden of care is shared. Such time- and energy-consuming clients are then cared for by team and congregation members, ensuring that no single individual burns out.

The AFCNA activated extra prayer support for clients, the FCNs, parish clergy, and health care chaplains. Various scientific and pastoral perspectives have noted the benefits of prayer (VandeCreek and Lyon, 1998; Carey, 2000b). For example, one FCN regularly visited newly released prisoners. She had three senior congregation members who prayed for her specific requests to ensure she could continue her work with such challenging clients. Confidentiality was always maintained, but this nurse found that the supplementary prayer sustenance enabled her to deal with several difficult client situations. All the FCNs in the demonstration project noted the importance of open times of shared prayer with the whole pastoral care team. Prayer created bonds between all the workers and helped to ensure the spiritual empowerment of the team to work together.

TRUST AND COMMUNICATION

Clear communication and good interpersonal skills are essential in creating a climate of trust. When FCNs speak to clergy in a direct and open manner, issues are dealt with before they become burdensome. Several clergy commented that they received additional support from the FCNs. One nurse stated she undertook "barometer checks" on her priest who was prone to overwork. She kept a regular check on his blood pressure and "body language." She watched for signs that he was getting "run down," recommending that he "take time off." He commented that he heeded her advice and felt that it improved his productivity and health.

All FCNs noted that they scheduled regular meetings with parish clergy to discuss confidentially plans, expectations, problems, and programs. They ran additional team meetings with pastoral care workers and health care chaplains, to plan, coordinate, delegate, discuss, and evaluate their work. An important factor in creating a positive team culture was receptivity to innovative ideas. Nurses have a unique perspective on many pastoral issues and most parish clergy found this refreshing and helpful. Mutual accountability about the various roles and functions of each team member ensured that the work was clearly defined, fairly delegated, and appropriately shared. One FCN noted that her team began each meeting with affirmations, each member stating something of value in the member's work in the past month. This prevented team meetings from focusing on problems and gripes. Instead of feeling burdened, the team left buoyed by the significance of their work. This same team also had a philosophy of praying if conflict or tension existed, committing these issues to prayer.

DEVELOPING A CONTINUUM OF SPIRITUAL CARE

Finally, the third significant collaboration involves the development of a continuum of spiritual care that includes health care chaplains, nurses, hospital-based health professionals, the congregational spiritual support team of the parish clergy, and FCNs. Australian health policy increasingly emphasizes the continuity of care along continuums that include primary, secondary, and tertiary health care providers. The church has a presence in all areas except primary health care, and FCN offers a significant opportunity to redress this deficit (Van Loon, 1998a). Research in Australia suggests that the majority of health care chaplains, through their respective pastoral care departments, have developed a valuable rapport with clinical staff, patients/clients, and their relatives (Carey, 1999a,b; Carey, 2000a). This research includes studies undertaken, for example, within organizations involving patients with cancer (Milne, 1988), pediatric conditions (Carey, 1995; Carey, Aroni, and Edwards, 1997), liver transplants (Elliot and Carey, 1996), brain injury (Ireland et al., 1999), and care for the aged (Mulder and Carey, 1999).

However, regardless of how well chaplains perform, growing economic pressure threatens universal health care in Australia and places increased strain on the demands of pastoral care departments. Changing trends mean that an increasing number of clients are in the hospital for a short duration, and this restricts the opportunity of health care chaplains to deal with long-term spiritual issues. It seems imperative that such patients receive a spiritual continuum of care alongside the physical and mental care components. The FCN model is uniquely designed to help address this issue.

Economic rationalism and the downsizing of some pastoral care departments also mean that chaplains have limited budgets as well as time. Health expenditure in Australia approximates 8.5 percent of the gross domestic product; expenditures average around $A2,294 per person per year for most of this decade (Australian Institute of Health and Welfare [AIHW], 1997b, p. 1). Several national health strategies over the past decade have sought to contain escalating costs. These include reorientation of mental health services, mainstreaming psychiatric care, increasing hostel accommodation for seniors, and decreasing nursing home beds by creating an "aging in place" policy, maintaining maximum bed occupancy in public hospitals, increasing day surgery, and reducing the length of stay of patients in tertiary facilities (AIHW, 1992, p. 121; AIHW, 1997a). When these facts are combined with an aging population and a contracting national tax base, the consequence of fiscal strain is a major concern. The taxpaying population is already under pressure from escalating Social Security payments to an aging population and from swelling ranks of the unemployed. These pressures particularly impact hospitals and elder care institutions.

The Australian government's response to this growing fiscal strain includes the encouragement of coordinated care. The World Bank (1993) itself encourages coordinated care in response to altered structures of payment for health care worldwide. The Australian government is introducing various forms of capitated care aimed at providing quality, cost-effective health care that is evidence based and outcomes oriented (Duckett, Hogan, and Southgate, 1995; Brand, 1996; Duckett, 1996). Policy shifts to address these issues have led to examination of client-focused models of care that measure productivity (Baldwin, 1994).

Introducing FCN into the continuum of health care meets these criteria and establishes the care continuum in the wider community. The current Australian health system focuses on physical repair of the body. People, however, are not machines that need to be repaired; they are relational beings. Given ailing government finances, the focus moves to crisis management. Chronically ill people oscillate between acute and chronic episodes of their disease. The government, recognizing its failure to manage chronic illness effectively, is using the national "coordinated care" trials to address the situation.

Modern medicine may cure the disease but leave the person un-healed. Conversely, some people with incurable disease are healed. From a religious perspective, healing is about restoring relationships within the individual, between people, the creation, and God. These reconciled relationships give a deep sense of inner peace, wholeness, and well-being (the Hebrews called it *shalom*). Thus, healing is in every sense a spiritual activity. God provides healing, and as God's servants, the faith community has a responsibility to be a healing center. Health care chaplains and FCNs can help to support this care by linking hospitals and parish clergy.

Bioethical issues also require a liaison between health care chaplains and faith communities. Research in Australian and New Zealand suggests that approximately 70.9 percent of Australian health and welfare chaplains and 57 percent of New Zealand inter-church council hospital chaplains are involved in bioethical decision making within their respective hospitals (Carey, Aroni, and Edwards, 1996; Carey, Aroni, and Gronlund, 1998). Lysaught (1994, 1998) strongly argues that one of the challenges of the church today is to engage in bioethical moral discourse and "to renew the congregation as the place where it occurs" (Lysaught, 1998, p. 558). For Lysaught, faith communities should not allow themselves to be designated as idiosyncratic groups whose religious convictions are incommensurate. The role of education and nurture in the development of values is integral to creating a framework for healthy living. Respect and love for the whole person should be value engendered and nurtured in any faith community (Van Loon, 1998b). Bioethical issues, even those as complex as genetic medicine, require discussion at the local church level; without such discussions congregants are "ill-equipped" and thus not in a position to make a "faithful" contribution to societal issues (Lysaught, 1998, p. 558). The education of congregations concerning bioethical issues is a particular continuum of spiritual care that FCNs can facilitate.

FCN AND CHAPLAINCY PILOT PROJECT

The first piloted attempt in Australia to create a complete model of continuum spiritual care that involved health care chaplains was undertaken in Sydney, New South Wales. The health care chaplains at

Sydney Adventist Hospital created an ecumenical regional network of FCNs based in faith communities around Sydney's North Shore region. Health care chaplains, nurses, and other health professionals have continued to supply tertiary spiritual support in the hospital and the secondary health services, while primary spiritual support and health care have been successfully provided in the faith community via the parish clergy and the FCNs. Evaluations of this continuum have been planned.

The predominate focus upon Adelaide (from where FCN initially developed) and Sydney are only two examples of FCN programs preparing and commencing in Australia. Since its inception, the AFCNA has actively promoted the FCN role and provided consultancy regarding the establishment of such ministries throughout Australia and New Zealand. FCN programs have now commenced in most Australian states and territories, and their role is drawing significant interest from government and health institutions (Table 12.2). Support of FCN is also proving to be ecumenical. FCN programs have thus far been sponsored or co-sponsored by Lutheran, Anglican, Catholic, Uniting, Baptist, Church of Christ, and Pentecostal churches.

EPILOGUE

The AFCNA is currently addressing challenges created by collaborations between parishes, parish clergy, chaplains, hospitals, doctors,

TABLE 12.2. Number of Faith Community Nurses by Region (Rank Order)

Region	Number of Faith Community Nurses
South Australia (SA)	28
Victoria (VIC)	10
New South Wales (NSW)	3
Queensland (Qld)	3
New Zealand (NZ)	3
Australian Capital Territory (ACT)	2
Western Australia (WA)	1
Northern Territory (NT)	0
Tasmania (TAS)	0

Source: Australian Faith Community Nurses Association.

nurses, allied health, and patients. Challenges include identifying the population to be served, interagency communication and referral systems, and identifying the responsibilities and the resources each faith community and hospital will bring to the relationship. Other issues include accountability and autonomy for the faith community, the role of hospital pastoral care departments, relationships with AFCNA, meeting nursing regulatory and legal statutory requirements, professional indemnity and public liability responsibilities, as well as communication across the collaboration continuum, including referral, confidentiality, and documentation.

Even given the vast amount of work to be undertaken and the necessary protocols to be established, the benefits of such a collaboration in Australia seem to be beneficial to all concerned. Further establishment of FCN programs in Australia will necessitate some form of national evaluation. Health care chaplains, in particular, given their training, experience, and rapport with medical and nursing professions, are vital to the enhancement of such a service and helpful in the long-term assessment and viability of FCN in Australia.

REFERENCES

Australian Bureau of Statistics (ABS) (1996). *Census of population and housing, 1911-1996.* Canberra, Australia: Australian Government Publishing Services.

Australian Faith Community Nurses Association (AFCNA) (1999a). *Faith community nursing and your church*: (video). Adelaide, South Australia: Author.

Australian Faith Community Nurses Association (AFCNA) (1999b). *Faith community nursing: A resource manual.* Adelaide, South Australia: Author.

Australian Institute of Health and Welfare (AIHW) (1992). *Australia's health 1992: The third biennial report of the Australian Institute of Health and Welfare.* Canberra, Australia: Australian Government Publishing Services.

Australian Institute of Health and Welfare (AIHW) (1997a). *Australian hospital statistics, 1995-96.* Canberra, Australia: Australian Government Publishing Services.

Australian Institute of Health and Welfare (AIHW) (1997b). *Health expenditure bulletin, No. 13.* Canberra, Australia: Australian Government Publishing Services.

Baldwin, R. (1994). *Managed care: A discussion paper.* Australian College of Health Care Executives, Vol. 4, No. 1. New South Wales, Sydney, Australia.

Brand, D. J. (1996). General practice reform: The shared management model. *Medical Journal of Australia,* 164(19), 221-223.

Carey, L.B. (1995). The role of chaplains: A research overview. *Ministry, Society and Theology, 9*(20), 41-53.

Carey, L.B. (1999a). *Chaplaincy in the clinical context: Anthology of published articles* (Volume 1). Melbourne, Australia: Australian Chaplaincy Utility Research.

Carey, L.B. (1999b). Health care chaplaincy research, *Journal of Family Studies, 5*(2), 291ff.

Carey, L.B. (2000a). Health care chaplaincy: A research snapshot. *Ministry Journal of Continuing Education, 10*(2), 28-30.

Carey, L.B. (2000b). Prayer in the clinical context. *Ministry, Society and Theology, 14*(1), 41-52.

Carey, L.B., Aroni, R., Edwards, A. (1996). Medical ethics and the role of hospital chaplains: A case study research report. *Ministry, Society and Theology, 10*(2), 66-79.

Carey, L.B., Aroni, R., and Edwards, A. (1997). Health policy and well-being: Hospital chaplaincy. In Gardner, H. (ed.) *Health policy in Australia.* Melbourne, Australia: Oxford University Press, pp. 190-210.

Carey, L.B., Aroni, R., and Gronlund, M. (1998). Bio-medical ethics, clinical decision making and hospital chaplaincy in New Zealand: A research progress report. *Ministry, Society and Theology, 12*(2), 136-156.

Duckett, S. J. (1996). Prospects for managed care in Australia. *Australian Health Review, 19*(2), 7-22.

Duckett, S.J., Hogan, T., and Southgate, J. (1995). The COAG reforms and community health services. *Australian Journal of Primary Health Interchange, 1*(1), 3-10.

Elliot, H. and Carey, L.B. (1996). The hospital chaplain's role in an organ transplant unit. *Ministry, Society and Theology, 10*(1), 66-77.

Granger, W. (1955). *Nurse, pastor, and patient.* Philadelphia, PA: Augsburg Fortress Press.

Hughes, P. (1999). Ministry in the Year of Older Persons. *Pointers, 9*(4), 1-5.

Hughes, P., Thompson, C., Pryor, R., and Bouma, G. (1995). *Believe it or not: Australian spirituality and the churches in the 90s.* Victoria, Australia: Christian Research Association.

Ireland, B., Carey, L.B., Baguley, I., Maurizi, R., Crooks, J., Gronlund, M. (1999). The Westmead Hospital Brain Injury Rehabilitation Unit and Pastoral Care Department pilot research project: A joint research endeavour. *Ministry, Society and Theology, 13*(1), 46-60.

Kaldor, P., Bellamy, J., Powell, R., Castle, K., and Hughes, B. (1999). *Build my church: Trends and possibilities for Australian churches.* Adelaide, Australia: National Church Life Survey, Open Book Publishers.

Kaldor, P., Bellamy, J., Powell, R., Correy, M., and Castle, K. (1994). *Winds of change: The experience of church in a changing Australia.* Sydney, Australia: National Church Life Survey, Homebush West, Lancer Books.

Kaldor, P., Bellamy, J., Powell, R., Hughes, B., and Castle, K. (1997). *Shaping a future: Characteristics of vital congregations.* Sydney, Australia: National Church Life Survey, Open Book Publishers.

Lysaught, M.T. (1994). From clinic to congregation: Religious communities and genetic medicine. *Christian Scholars Review, 23*(3), 329-348.

Lysaught, M.T. (1998). From clinic to congregation. In Lammers, S. and Verhey, A. (eds.) (1998), *On moral medicine: Theological perspectives in medical ethics* (Second edition), Cambridge, UK: Eerdmans Publishing, pp. 547-561.

Milne, J. (1988). Patients' and their families' reflections on pastoral care in their cancer experience—Report of a survey. *Cancer Forum, 12*(3), 115-123.

Mulder, C. and Carey, L.B. (1999). Our Lady of Consolation aged care services—Results and critique of a pilot pastoral care resident's survey. *Ministry, Society and Theology, 13*(2), 22-35.

Van Loon, A.M. (1998a). The development of faith community nursing programs as a response to changing Australian health policy. *Health Education and Behaviour, 25*(6), 790-799.

Van Loon, A.M. (1998b). Respect, love and the need to care: A triad which keeps nurses caring. In Nurses for Life South Australia (eds.), *Nurses for life, bioethics and related issues.* Adelaide, Australia: Open Book Publishers.

Van Loon, A.M. (1999). Creating a conceptual model of faith community nursing in Australia using participatory action research. PhD thesis dissertation. Adelaide, South Australia: Flinders University.

VandeCreek, L. and Lyon, M.A. (1998). Ministry of hospital chaplains: Patient satisfaction. *Journal of Health Care Chaplaincy, 6*(2), 1-59.

Westberg, G.E. (1989). Parish nursing pioneer. *The Journal of Christian Nursing, 6*(1), 26-29.

Westberg, G.E. (1990). A historical perspective: Wholistic health and the parish nurse. In Solari-Twadell, P.A., Djupe, A.M., and McDermott, M.A. (Eds.), *Parish nursing: The developing practice* (pp. 27-39). Park Ridge, IL: Lutheran General Health System.

Westberg, G.E. and Westberg McNamara, J. (1990). *The parish nurse: Providing a minister of health for your congregation.* Minneapolis, MN: Augsburg Fortress Press.

World Bank (1993). *World development report 1993: Investing in health.* Oxford, UK: Oxford University Press.

SECTION V:
PRACTICE MODELS

Chapter 13

A Parish Nurse and Pastor Reflect on the Personal and Corporate Ministry of Pastoral Care

William R. Leety
Sue Mooney

Overbrook Presbyterian Church is an 800-member congregation with a professional staff of two ordained clergy, a full-time minister of music, and a part-time volunteer parish nurse. The church also sponsors a preschool program. In this chapter, we describe the parish nurse program, including some of our theological and organizational assumptions about it.

MINISTRY IS PERSONAL, CORPORATE, AND COLLABORATIVE

Congregation and staff intend pastoral care and health ministry to provide a personal, corporate ministry. It is personal. Each provider and recipient of pastoral care has a face and story, a unique place in the congregation, and a call to ministry. It is corporate. Pastoral care and the nurture of personal health, whether of members or the larger community, is an expression of the whole. Care offered to one is care for the whole.

Congregation and staff take family and family systems theory seriously, proclaiming and practicing the self-definition of "family." A widow living alone, except for memories of a spouse, and whose children are at a distance is by self-definition a family. Parents plus child (even if the child is fifty-five years old) sharing an apartment is a family. The last living member of an entire family residing in the nursing home is by self-definition a family.

Pastoral care recognizes "personal" history (or story) and preference. Nearly everyone relates more easily, or at least differently, to women and to men. Consequently, sometimes a female clergy takes the lead in providing care to selected families. Sometimes a male clergy is the professional of choice. Some members of the congregation have a history with other members or with staff. There can be decades of shared story, celebrated joys, or notorious distress and distrust. For instance, members Les and Marty (pseudonyms) got close when Les's first wife was sick; Charlene and Judy were on different sides when the congregation was deciding whether to dismiss Pastor Marsden. People in the congregation may feel close or distant with one member of staff or another. As partners with members of a congregation, everyone must take seriously relationships such as they are.

"You can't help who you like," Robin's grandmother used to say. People are drawn to some and not to others. Affection and love are mysterious, as is absence of affection: "I just can't make myself like him." Therefore, when people hurt, they want someone's hand, not anyone's, holding theirs. They want some listener, not any listener, to hear them tell their story of surgery and ask, "Why has God let me live to be so old?" There is a particular person with a name given in baptism whose prayers they covet.

If members cannot help their affection for staff members, deacons, or Stephen Ministers, neither can staff make themselves fond of all recipients of care. However, staff must recognize their affections or lack thereof, and act in the best interest and for the well-being of the person, sometimes because the staff member is the only one in the room with that member at the time. Sometimes deep crevices in relationships are filled in during times of illness.

Congregations are multilingual, not only in formal language, e.g., Spanish or Swahili, but also in the dialects of disciplines and generations. As at Pentecost, different tongues of fire appear on different heads. Now the Spirit works to bring mutual understanding. Consequently, this congregation deliberately engages staff members who speak different dialects. A parish nurse speaks medicine and theology and insurance. A parish associate speaks and understands therapeutic accents. In specific situations of pastoral care, one dialect may be more helpful than another.

Congregations are organic; they move and mutate, breathe and decline. Together the members are entrusted with the ministry of Christ. Some members are set apart for particular ministries of care, such as deacons, Stephen Ministers, and parish nurses. Still, each Christian inevitably confronts the question, "Who is my neighbor?" So, while particular members or staff may be set apart as providers of pastoral care, they minister on behalf of the whole. In this congregation, members, though not set apart by ordination or special gifts, often lead ministries of pastoral care because of their strong relationships to the receivers of care. In these instances, staff are advised and invited into secondary roles to provide support to lay caregivers. For instance, as Mark got close to Carl during Carl's last months, he would check with the parish nurse: "Do you think he needs to see the doctor, or is this normal for a man so sick?" Jane called to say, "When I had surgery, Doris was so helpful. Now that Pete's having that same surgery, how do you think I can be his 'Doris'?" Staff most frequently encourage Jane and Mark to "wade in." People of faith can support one another in ways only God knows.

WELLNESS AND ILLNESS

"In sickness and in health" is a key element in wedding vows; yet sickness and health happen to all. In a collaborative style of health ministry and pastoral care, it is important that staff share broad theological understandings about illness and health. Members of this staff begin with Job—health and illness are mysterious. When caregivers must choose whether to speak from the perspective of God or from the perspective of the one who is suffering, they should, unlike Job's friends, choose the perspective of the suffering. This staff shares the conviction of the apostle, loosely paraphrased, "nothing can separate us from the love of God . . . neither Alzheimer's nor AIDS, neither bipolar disorder nor colon cancer, neither the current mutation of flu nor narcolepsy . . . nothing in all creation can separate us from the love of God."

This staff does not have major theological differences on the issue of health, such as whether illness or death is God's punishment for sin. (Granted that if Fred keeps eating sausage, he may develop clogged arteries, and if Alice continues smoking, her cardiovascular system will suffer and perhaps bring her down to death—nonetheless, people do not need a God to damn them or bring death. Of that, people are capable on their own.) This staff affirms that "there's a time to be born and a time to die"—every birth certificate contains metaphorical fine print that reads "you shall also die." And with the apostle Paul, staff believe that death and life are a bigger deal to humans than to God—"If we live, we live to the Lord and if we die, we die to the Lord; so whether we live or whether we die, we are the Lord's." In any case, really *any* case, a giver of pastoral care is to side with the sufferer and let God take care of God's own self. It's fine to say, "If you continue this high-risk behavior you'll get AIDS." But, it is not fine to say so without adding, "and I don't want that to happen. But if it does I'll stand or sit with you."

At issue in health ministry are, simultaneously, the wholeness of persons and the wholeness of community. For example, a person needs meals and transportation arranged when and after leaving the hospital. The congregation, to remember its identity, may share responsibility for a discharge plan with the person leaving the hospital and with the person's family.

Although illness is an ordinary human experience, it raises issues of faith, hope and love, and ultimate questions:

- Am I in communion or alone?
- Who am I . . . without my activity? without my prostate or breast or energy or fetus? my good humor or voice? Am I loved, loveable?
- Am I only spirit? Or, am I body, corporeal, carnal, flesh?

How a person answers these fundamental questions and lives may contribute toward *sickness or health.* Clues to answers often come in honest interaction with others. For example, when Jesus was distressed, someone anointed his feet. Touched by the anointing, Jesus predicted, "What she has done will be remembered." So, touch and food and words are remembered and identify the community of caregivers, while also serving the distressed or ill.

At the least, illness renders a person, and sometimes even the community of whom that person is a part, vulnerable or afraid. Illness can be occasion for discovery or growth or loss of faith, or simultaneous discovery and loss. Pastoral caregivers minister to persons, families, and the community. Staff resources of time and expertise are allocated on the principle that when choices must be made about whose needs are served, the most vulnerable person comes first.

STAFF FOR PASTORAL CARE—AS ART

In this congregation, parish nursing works as an indispensable part of *health* ministry. Though there is a design, it is difficult to say whether parish nursing and health ministry work *by* design or *despite* design.

"Staff" is comprised of people monetarily compensated and uncompensated, full- and part-time, and "recruited volunteers"—persons invited for specific gifts they bring. Staff understand themselves as parts of a team or "body," whether members of the congregation or other congregations, or nonmembers. They function as an "interprofessional team," defined a quarter century ago as

> a small, organized group of persons, each trained in different professional disciplines and possessing unique skills and orientations, among whom there is an organized division of labor, around a common problem, with each member contributing his [*sic*] own talents, with continuous intercommunication, re-examination and re-evaluation of individual efforts in terms of the limitations provided by team goals and objectives, and with group responsibility for the final outcome. (Kane, 1975, p. 3)

The management model employed with staff is aesthetic. Simply put, the task is to produce the "prettiest picture" within the limits of the resources of congregation and staff. Responsibility falls upon staff and congregation both as individuals and as a collective (Siehl, 1978). On any given day resources may be monochromatic—one crayon available—or polychromatic—two crayons "in the box." On a great day this congregation has more than two talented professionals at hand.

Despite daily changes of resources, routine is established. Parish nurse, pastor, and parish associates are assigned to hospital visits one day each week. Sometimes the minister of music is included in the rotation. On weekends a pastor or parish associate is on call, supplemented by the parish nurse.

Records are maintained. Visits with those in hospital and residents of care institutions and rehabilitation centers are charted. Staff record their perceptions for the benefit of other staff, both as comparison and as preparation for a next visit. Each staff member reports monthly to the governing board the number and kind of interactions with congregation members and with community members who seek the services of the church (e.g., hospital and home visits, follow-up contacts postdischarge from hospital, counseling appointments, contacts at blood pressure screenings).

At a weekly meeting, staff discuss specific people who are suffering, just as nurses and physicians pass information and perceptions at the change of shifts for those in their care. The assignment for a next call is made or a plan for continuing outreach is developed. A plan may include building a network of care in which other church members share responsibility. In this process confidences are kept, and assessments are shared visitor to visitor. The staff also share views to discern the person's theology of his or her illness, e.g., anger at God, an occasion for God's glory.

Support staff members participate in the conversations at staff meetings. They are frequently the initial contact for hurting people. They also provide added eyes, ears, and insights into the stories of people a church staff collaboratively serves. People who are ill or well relate differently to different staff. For example, when the parish nurse visits, Lee may always seem energetic and upbeat, and when the pastor visits, Lee may always seem complaining and depressed. Shared perceptions allow the parish nurse to suggest during a visit, "The pastor thought you seemed sad. I hadn't sensed that on my visits. Do you think you're depressed?" Sometimes members, in the course of conversation about meetings or schedules, speak with the office manager of illness or wellness in themselves or others in the congregation. A weekly meeting provides an opportunity to apply the collective experiences of staff to serve the congregation. The parish nurse brings competence about medical issues that informs other staff about the broader issues faced by members. When requested or judged appropriate, two or more staff together may visit a person who is ill. Occasionally these visits are quasi-interventions.

The staff maintain no "hierarchy" of visits to sick or homebound members. The day of the week on which the church learns of the admission dictates which staff person visits first. On occasion, a specific staff person is requested for a specific situation. For example, a person in hospice may say, "When my children come next week, I want the pastor and minister of music to visit, so that we can plan my funeral." A person recovering from surgery may tell the pastor, "I'd like to see the parish nurse a day or two before I'm discharged to talk about aftercare for an ostomy." As a matter of course, staff members refer individuals to other staff and to nonstaff. On discovering that Bill, a person undergoing dialysis, appreciates glass paperweights, a staff person invites Maxine, a lifelong collector of paperweights, to show him several in her collection. On learning of Pat's need for rehab services, a parish associate or pastor asks, "May I share what you've told me with the parish nurse? Our nurse has lived in the city a long time and been involved in public health and visiting care institutions more than I." The continuing question before staff is, "How can this church do the best job with and for this member, this family?" Issues of staff egos, should they arise, are dealt with apart from issues of pastoral care.

This congregation and staff benefit from church relationships with a seminary and a nursing school. Each year student nurses and student pastors work with church staff in pastoral care. Their fresh ears and eyes give the regular staff insights into how "an outsider" perceives the pastoral care ministry and help ascertain nearsightedness or distorted vision.

Wellness ministries are sometimes done jointly by staff. Pastor and parish nurse together counsel with a pregnant couple preparing for marriage and parenthood, or with a couple considering genetic or fertility testing, or with a single woman considering working with a sperm bank to bear a child. The volunteer coordinator and parish associate together assist newly retired or laid-off workers to use their available time productively. The parish nurse and pastor counsel with families making medical care decisions, such as establishing medical power of attorney, giving advance directives, or considering organ donation. They advocate for families concerning issues of insurance and plans for discharge. Inevitably church staff and selected congregational members know the homes to which hospitalized persons return better than the employees of health care institutions who develop discharge plans. The pastoral care staff believe that no person hospitalized should be without a health care advocate.

The congregation also uses staff in more public settings of pastoral care. Frequently the parish nurse assists in leading worship at services of witness to the resurrection (funerals). Her long tenure in the community and church allows the parish nurse to offer continuity of care at this important public occasion. Pastors, the nurse, and deacons gather members of families bereaved during the past year before year-end holidays to think together about "this first Christmas," and to remember "last" holidays and other anniversaries. The best gifts and wisdom at these gatherings are brought by the bereaved themselves as they share experiences since the death and think together about celebrating these holy days faithfully.

The parish nurse may also serve as "worship leader" in other circumstances. Customarily the nurse prays with members whom she visits or counsels. She or others of the staff may use a liturgy of anointing. She may serve as "assisting elder or deacon" when the Lord's Supper is served to persons homebound or hospitalized. Word, sacrament, and service are joined.

The specific duties of the parish nurse in pastoral care match her gifts and professional education:

- Blood pressure screening the second Sunday of each month between services of worship, and at Christian education intergeneration learning events
- Informing the congregation of and publicizing other health screenings, e.g., mammograms, prostate cancer screenings
- Providing information regarding prescription and over-the-counter medicines, diet supplements, and alternative therapies
- Assisting in sponsoring blood donor drives
- Arranging vision and hearing screening for children in the church's weekday preschool, and providing follow-up for early intervention
- Serving as referral for preschool students with special needs

- Teaching church and preschool staff (and parents) cardiopulmonary resuscitation
- Teaching health education to preschoolers

In summary, parish nursing always takes place within the contexts of human relationships and theological assumptions embodied in the congregation and the church staff members. We have sought to demonstrate how, within one congregation, parish nursing is an essential part of our ministry. Ministry, from our perspective, is personal, corporate, and collaborative.

REFERENCES

Kane, R. (1975). *Interprofessional teamwork.* Syracuse, NY: Division of Continuing Education and Manpower, Syracuse University School of Social Work.

Siehl, J. C. (1978). An investigation of the effects of an interprofessional health care course on student attitudes. Unpublished thesis. Columbus: The Ohio State University, p. 12.

Chapter 14

A Conversation with Pastoral Church Staff Members About Their Parish Nurse Program

Pastoral Staff of the Overbrook Presbyterian Church,
Columbus, Ohio

This edited telephone interview elaborates on the parish nursing program described in the previous chapter by involving other staff members in the discussion. They talk with the interviewer about the history of the program, its theological foundations, how they relate to one another as staff members, and how the program functions within the context of the congregation.

INTERVIEWER: I think it would be helpful if one of you would begin by describing the congregation and the professional staff.

PASTOR: We are a metropolitan congregation of eight hundred members in a large city. Our neighborhood is a couple of miles north of a major university and we are probably a bit older and better educated than the general population of the city. Forty percent of our members live within a one-mile radius in the church. We have a weekday preschool that sometimes becomes engaged in issues of health ministry. Our professional staff includes a full-time director of the preschool, a full-time minister of music, two part-time parish associates, a parish nurse, and myself as pastor. Support staff in the office includes an administrative manager, an office manager, and volunteers from the congregation.

PARISH NURSE: I think that it's important that we do serve the city; we have city problems and city issues. For awhile, I think the congregation saw itself as a suburban church but we really are a city church.

PASTOR: That is one of the qualities of the staff here; we tend to agree that there are two definitions of our parish. There is the older geographic one that says we are on a specific corner in this neighborhood. The other definition consists of membership rolls. I believe the staff here tends to work from both those definitions.

INTERVIEWER: Perhaps the next step could be to describe how the parish nurse program began.

PARISH NURSE: Actually, it began on two levels. Our congregation suffered a lot of conflict in the preceding decade and we began to look at how that was happening. We began to talk about what the church would look like if we were to include a wellness ministry as a mission focus. We wanted to change perceptions among the membership that, rather than a place of brokenness, the church was a place of healing. We had experienced a lot of brokenness and it seemed like this was a good time to begin to look at how we might change that. On a second level, I was volunteer coordinator in the congregation at that time and the staff became increasingly aware that my work was more nursing oriented. The question arose as to whether we should change the focus of my role to that of a parish nurse rather than that of volunteer coordinator.

INTERVIEWER: So the program began in part because the volunteer coordinator was a nurse?

PASTOR: I believe there were other factors too. Our volunteer coordinator was a nurse but also an ordained elder, and the year the parish nurse program began, she was elected moderator of the presbytery.

INTERVIEWER: So this was a situation in which she was a known quantity. She had a history in the congregation.

PASTOR: She was known as a church person. In some situations it is important to ask the parish nurse, "Do you work for the health care provider system or do you work for the church?" From the beginning, that question was already explicitly answered. She had credibility as a church person.

INTERVIEWER: So did the parish nurse program begin during the tenure of the current pastor?

PARISH NURSE: No, he came into it unaware of what he was getting into.

INTERVIEWER: How has that gone?

PASTOR: I think it has gone rather smoothly. I never had a parish nurse on staff before. Given my experience here, it would be hard for me to lead a church staff without one. I have done discharge planning in three previous parishes and I had nurse friends in the parish who helped me not mess up too badly. The parish nurse program was in place when I came here, and my understanding of the call is to get along with the staff who are already present. And if the pastor-elect can't buy that part of the call then that's not a helpful call. Part of the task is simply to come and be a part of the team that is already in place.

INTERVIEWER: Certainly not to fire everyone who is there and bring your own team in.

PASTOR: In my judgment, that is against the rules, against the way God works.

INTERVIEWER: This is a good place to transition to a serious question that needs wider discussion. From your perspective, what are the theological underpinnings of the parish nurse program and, as you experience it, how does theology influence it? There is a wide diversity of theology, of course, across these programs and I would be interested in hearing you talk about yours.

FIRST PARISH ASSOCIATE: The tone is set by the pastor, the session, and the staff. In this staff and congregation, it's a very positive holistic approach to ministry, very broad, and the trust level is built in and it develops over time.

INTERVIEWER: So the playing field is level; each participant is equal?

FIRST PARISH ASSOCIATE: Yes, and it works very smoothly here in my observation because, first of all, pastoral care is a priority. Second, it works because of the expectations of the congregation. Third, it works because of the caring personality of the parish nurse, and, fourth, it works because of the respect the staff has for one another's talents, experiences, and disciplines.

INTERVIEWER: Any other theological underpinnings that you want to mention?

SECOND PARISH ASSOCIATE: I think one of the theological underpinnings is the notion of healing. Jesus was engaged in a healing ministry and certainly reflected a very holistic viewpoint. I think that Jesus touched many different aspects of the human being, their social, physical, mental, and spiritual health, certainly. I think that healing is certainly a biblical theology concept. I also believe that the theological concept of hospitality is important, the kind of hospitality in which we go out to meet others in their need. We invite people to the church, of course, and we include them in our community when they come. This obviously involves healing. But then we also go outward to meet others in our pastoral care efforts. That certainly supports the idea of parish nursing.

INTERVIEWER: Would one of you talk about "care" as a pervasive concept within the church that, in turn, I assume is one of the theological motivations for parish nursing?

FIRST PARISH ASSOCIATE: I would offer a rather unique perspective because I experienced this parish nursing program as a staff colleague and as a patient. When I had a serious cancer surgery, this parish nurse was my friend, was a professional, and was part of the same parish staff as myself. Even when I was unconscious in intensive care, she was, unbeknownst to me, advocating for me. Later during my recovery, I confided some intimate things about my procedure and recovery to her. So I experienced the parish nurse as a patient and then as a colleague.

INTERVIEWER: That is a reflection not just on your experience as a professional but also as a person.

FIRST PARISH ASSOCIATE: Exactly!

PASTOR: In the biblical literature, it seems that illness is often perceived as a boundary that cuts people off from community. That was a problem for Jesus, and he made problems for others when he invited people in. There are all sorts of rituals in first-century Judaism that caused illness to be a problem. It seems to me that the whole Bible takes seriously that we're going to die someday; the length of life is limited. It also takes seriously that illness is mysterious to some degree. It's not very mysterious if you smoke cigarettes; bad things can happen to you. But, it's still mysterious. It's a common human experience and Jesus dealt with it hospitably and seemed to say that we ought to reach out to people who are experiencing poor health.

INTERVIEWER: So you disagree with the view that sickness is a result of specific sins.

SECOND PARISH ASSOCIATE: It seems to me, that was the notion of sin in Judaism and in the New Testament. If you were ill, you must have done something sinful to cause that.

PASTOR: I believe the story of Job in the Old Testament says that if you must choose between the afflicted person and God, your responsibility is toward the afflicted person rather than God.

INTERVIEWER: We should transition now to why and how the parish nurse program works. One concern that appears repeatedly in literature concerns the use of authority, status, and responsibility. In other words, who has the most authority? Who has the responsibility and how is it shared? Much of this has to do with defining and maintaining professional boundaries. What could happen among yourselves that would make you nervous about your professional boundaries?

FIRST PARISH ASSOCIATE: I think that we are all aware of the limits of our talents and knowledge. That is unique to this staff. We like, respect, and trust each other and I have not experienced any conflict at all here. I think we have exemplary staff relationships. I have felt complete openness with staff, and I think this emanates from the pastor's own attitude. That attitude is the foundation of how we relate to each other and the congregation.

INTERVIEWER: So there is a considerable amount of permission giving on the part of the pastor.

PARISH NURSE: I think one of the keys is the very open communication that goes on here. Staff members are always available to each other and there are no stated limits as to what any of us can or cannot do in providing pastoral care. If I visit someone that I think would benefit from a visit from another staff member, I talk with the pastor and then talk with the staff member. We can call each other at home; there are no boundaries on that. If I am making visits and feel that I need help, I contact someone on the phone very quickly. I have never had a staff member refuse to come to my rescue on any problem, and this open communication and eagerness for each other to succeed is what makes it work.

PASTOR: One concrete example of that open communication is the pastoral care log that we keep as a staff. Like a hospital chart, we record our impressions after a visit so that other staff members can build on that in subsequent visits. An individual congregant might have a visit from a different staff member four times in one week, but each staff member is informed by previous visits.

PARISH NURSE: I want to make clear that we don't share information with another staff member unless we have asked permission from the congregant. I will say, "Is it okay if I share this with the other staff?" I always have their verbal permission. For me, the surprising response from almost everyone is that they are pleased and reassured that the staff is concerned about them and working together to help them through this difficult time. There seems to be such genuine appreciation for the fact that staff is working together on their problems. When I do one of these follow-up visits, I will say, "The staff wanted me to visit you today. We were concerned about you yesterday." It is also important to note that the congregation seems to appreciate the different gifts that each of us brings to individual situations. We don't duplicate each other; we bring our individuality.

PASTOR: We visit parishioners in the local hospitals five days per week when we have our customary full staff. These visits rotate through the staff. When I visit on Tuesday, I will say to the parishioners that an associate will see them tomorrow. This lets parishioners know how we do business; they know that we do it together as a staff.

SECOND PARISH ASSOCIATE: That might lead to another oblique theological point, which is the whole idea of hope. When one staff member promises a visit the next day, the parishioner has something to hold on to. Someone will come the next day; that helps people in their outlook and promotes hope.

INTERVIEWER: They have something to anticipate.

FIRST PARISH ASSOCIATE: My understanding is that the reason the church employs us is to do the best job we can for the parish. They want us to do the best job collectively as a staff given the limits of our gifts. When one of us fails, corporately we fail. When one of us succeeds, corporately we succeed. We are responsible enough to one another that if we are not doing a good job with a situation, we tell the other one, "I am not doing a good job here. *Help!*"

INTERVIEWER: So you experience the freedom to call for help.

FIRST PARISH ASSOCIATE: Sure. We compare our impressions. "I think this person is depressed, how come you don't think so?" "I don't think this person is depressed, why are we treating her as though she were?"

INTERVIEWER: Are there boundaries between you all? Or are you duplicates of each other, with some of you having more gifts in one area than another?

PASTOR: I am sure we're not clones, but there are no set rules. I think that the trust level is so explicit with us that we just feel that. That seems implicit within this staff. I am sure that it is not possible to do this in every staff, but we have been able to do it here.

INTERVIEWER: Do you think that some characteristics of the congregation contribute to your ability as a staff to function in this way?

PASTOR: Certainly, and one of those characteristics is that we have multiple people with evident talents. Sometimes, as a staff we will say, "I think Tom or Jane who are parishioners could be helpful with this parishioner. Let's get them involved."

PARISH NURSE: We are never hesitant to draw on the gifts within the congregation. If we feel a member of the congregation can be helpful, we ask them to become involved.

FIRST PARISH ASSOCIATE: I think our music director/organist goes above and beyond what is ordinarily expected.

PARISH NURSE: It's not uncommon for him to make a hospital call.

FIRST PARISH ASSOCIATE: He really follows through and will seek out people and knows what is going on their lives. I've been really impressed with how he does that.

SECOND PARISH ASSOCIATE: He has known people for years and people have lots of affection for him and he for them. We trade on that.

PASTOR: The parish nurse sometimes gets calls to pray when someone dies either at home or in the hospital and that's okay. Sometimes she participates in funerals. People say it's really great to have a two-pastor funeral. Sometimes that happens here, not only two pastors but also two pastors and a parish nurse.

SECOND PARISH ASSOCIATE: These are corporate occasions and frequently the leadership expresses relationships throughout the church and the staff.

FIRST PARISH ASSOCIATE: I think that the pastor oversees the whole process and makes sure that these things happen. We always have a time in the staff meeting in which we talk about people. I think this needs to be mentioned because I've been on other staffs where this isn't intentionally done.

SECOND PARISH ASSOCIATE: The pastor does a lot of the calling himself. He is not only a preaching pastor.

INTERVIEWER: Let's shift the conversation now to the specific things that the parish nursing program accomplishes.

PARISH NURSE: I think of it as a public health ministry within a faith community. Let me name some of the things that I do. I organize health fairs. I oversee Red Cross blood drives. Flu immunizations will be done this fall. There is a preschool eye test coming up. At the moment, the children's health insurance program is taking up a tremendous amount of my time. It impacts the community even though that doesn't necessarily impact a lot of the children in the congregation. I am trying to raise the wellness committee's conscience level about this program. I am working with discharge planners at the hospital when a member is going home or to a special care facility. I know every pharmacist in this area of the city; they also have concerns for our members. Visiting in nursing homes, I am concerned that patients are being taken care of properly. I have developed relationships with the nursing home administrators, so they see me not as a snooper, but as someone that is on the team helping to take care of the members.

PASTOR: That is where the issue of whom you work for matters. The members of the parish understand that she works for God and for them.

PARISH NURSE: Suppose we stopped ten members of the congregation and asked, "What is a parish nurse or what does your parish nurse in your church do?" We would probably get ten very different answers because my ministry differs with what their needs are. With some people, it is mainly a presence, the advocacy role; sometimes it's taking lunch to someone. The other day I took lunch to a woman who loves Chinese food and is not able to leave her home and we ate together. Not exactly a nurse's function, yet while I was there I was able to assess how she is doing in her home.

FIRST PARISH ASSOCIATE: Part of the helpfulness here is being in someone's home. When one of us visits in someone's home for half an hour, we know more than we would have than if they had come to the office a dozen times.

PARISH NURSE: A few years ago the general assembly [United Presbyterian Church—USA] encouraged churches to form care teams
to work with HIV persons. Now the general assembly says, "Let's
see what we can do to expand that care team concept." As we were
talking about it, I began to see all kinds of areas where we really do
form care teams already. I was thinking of the care teams for an
older member we know pretty well. We formed a team when she
broke her hip and needed assisted-living care. Her apartment
needed to be taken apart, and we called in very qualified people in
the congregation who were very organized and knew how to do
this kind of thing. That team went in and cleaned the apartment,
sorted through her things, and helped her decide what things
needed to be discarded and what needed to go with her. A group of
people came in and actually did the move. Another person on the
team with great financial skills worked out the fiscal arrangements
for the care center. An attorney and member of the congregation
drew up her will and worked out power of attorney. This was a care
team. This was a group of people coming together to give specialized care to a person in the congregation.

INTERVIEWER: We need to be finishing in a moment. Are there other
things you want to say?

PASTOR: Thank you for this opportunity; this was an interesting opportunity. I have also felt edified by the helpful discussions we had
in preparation for this interview.

SECOND PARISH ASSOCIATE: One of the ways people know about parish nursing here at the church is the bulletin board that contains all
sorts of screenings and opportunities, which encourages people. I
have asked several people, "What makes parish nursing work in
this congregation?" They say it is the relationship they have with
the nurse.

INTERVIEWER: The character style of the nurse becomes very important. Of course the character style of everyone on the teams is very
important.

PASTOR: I think this is true about other advocates we have. For example, most people hire an attorney based on what they think about the
attorney's character.

INTERVIEWER: Anything else?

SECOND PARISH ASSOCIATE: I think parish nursing is a lot like social work because the program carries out many tasks that social workers have historically performed. I think the parish nurse goes beyond traditional nursing, although maybe not public health nursing. Public health nursing is an outreach. A care team in a congregation is like a case management team in mental health. A lot of different professionals come together, although one person heads the team and coordinates activities. Case management is really big in mental health now.

INTERVIEWER: I believe that is true. One of the differences is that when parish nurses carry out these tasks, they are not nearly as rule bound in terms of how many people have to be seen today.

PARISH NURSE: Very true. And I don't have the bureaucracy of third-party payments.

INTERVIEWER: Are there other things you wish to say? [After silence] I have the impression that we have covered the subject as we intended. I thank you for being part of this and wish you well.

Chapter 15

Connections, Collisions, and Complementarity: The Dynamic of Health Care Chaplain, Parish Nurse, and Parish Clergy Collaboration

Renae Schumann
Tim VanDuivendyk

BACKGROUND

This chapter describes a practice model in which parish nurses, health care chaplains, and community clergy collaborate to create communities of wholeness. The model exists in a multifacility, not-for-profit, interfaith-based health care system that draws from and supports community resources such as faith congregations. The system has an active chaplaincy and clinical pastoral education (CPE) program with at least one staff chaplain at each hospital. One full-time director of the extensive parish nurse program (congregational outreach program, or COP) assists area churches in developing programs and in recruiting and training congregation volunteers, usually registered nurses, to provide health and wellness education based on congregational need.

Chaplains and the COP director, who is a parish nurse, have many opportunities to interface with faith communities, especially with community clergy and parish nurses. They each experience a call to unique ministry and are each compelled to help people be better, feel better, and carry suffering better. They discipline themselves within their respective ministries to develop their professional knowledge, talents, and skills. Their relationship, however, is also the context for collisions and conflicts regarding care roles, boundaries, and priorities. If unresolved these lead to isolation, creating a negative and potentially detrimental situation for all involved. Connections can bring enjoyable and productive complementarity with energy and synergy for their mission.

CHAPLAIN AND PARISH NURSE
ENTRY INTO COMMUNITY

As health care professionals, chaplains and parish nurses share the mission of healthy, whole, and integrated communities without walls. Chaplains work primarily within the hospital setting but may team with community clergy and have connections within several congregational communities. Parish nurses may work within one or more parishes as well as in another field of nursing. Working toward this mission without walls requires chaplains and parish nurses to minister within the traditional healing community of the hospital, and to involve congregations and communities outside the hospital.

The Community Clergy Enter

Today, community clergy increasingly are asked to consider their role within parish health or healing ministries. Recognition of the effects of spiritual health and well-being on the whole person leads to the consideration of the church as a therapeutic community that carries the healing principles of religion and spirituality (Evans, 1999). In prior centuries the church had this healing role that has now been assumed by other institutions. Community clergy who are effective in general ministry are more likely to be sought after as healers by parishioners because healing is a part of general ministry. Parishioners who have enjoyed the benefits of spiritual health and healing as experienced within the therapeutic faith community are more likely to refer others from the general community to experience its caring aspects.

As community clergy become more involved in and familiar with the notion of healing, health, or caring ministries, they become more interested in expanding the programs of their congregations. As a result, a parish nurse is often included in the pastoral staff. The needs and resources of the congregation and the community define the parish nurse function and lay the foundation for a mission statement or plan. This statement can address issues of availability and competence in dealing with the needs and concerns of people (Nelson, 1999). It can encourage the congregation and community to participate in the health ministry by serving others who are suffering (Schumann, 1999). In an effort to fulfill the new mission, community clergy may interface with the health care system, especially with hospital chaplains and hospital-based parish nurse programs.

Collaboration in Community

In their pursuit of healthier and therapeutic communities, chaplains, parish nurses, and parish clergy collaborate in a number of activities designed to address community needs. They have many opportunities to complement and connect their practice skills, knowledge, and gifts. However, inherent in any collaboration are times when ministry patterns and philosophies can collide and, hopefully, achieve eventual complementarity as these differences in care goals are worked through and synergized.

DEFINITIONS AND CASE EXAMPLES

Connections

Connections occur as members from each field come together for the purpose of achieving a specified goal, such as a healthier community. Parties within the connecting team bring their individual calls to ministry, professional knowledge, talents, skills, and missions. The collaborative practice model described within this section was initiated and became successful by using a number of these connections.

When this COP was started, the hospital system consisted of six acute care facilities. The COP director was responsible for implementing the program in each of the hospitals and formed a steering committee, composed of one representative from each hospital and serving as an advisory board to the COP director. Committee members were familiar with the politics and environments of their individual hospitals and were therefore able to facilitate successful program establishment.

Each steering committee member was chair of a COP subcommittee at his or her respective hospital, members of which were recommended by the steering committee and the hospital chaplain. These subcommittees were composed of the chaplain and other hospital employees, area community clergy, area parish nurses, and, in some cases, area business leaders. In no instances were the clergy and the parish nurses from the same congregation. Whereas the steering committee was familiar with the hospitals, the subcommittees were familiar with the communities.

Each subcommittee advised the COP director regarding the needs of that hospital's service area and helped initiate programs intended to meet those needs. Hospital chaplains, parish nurses, and community clergy collaborated toward the common goal of healthier communities. Community clergy and parish nurses serving on the subcommittees were proactive in establishing health programs within their own congregations, and they learned how to utilize the services of the hospital and the community to provide quality care. Other hospital employees and business leaders serving on the committee also became interested in congregational health and introduced the idea to their respective congregation leaders.

Collaborative efforts produced a system of preventive health care, including newsletters, cardiopulmonary resuscitation (CPR) classes, ongoing health education, support groups, health fairs, and many other congregation-specific programs that were supported by the congregations, the area hospitals, and the community. As the COP and individual congregational programs grew and strengthened, hospital chaplains, community clergy, and parish nurses helped and advised one another, often crossing denominational and geographic boundaries.

Collisions

Connections also bring collisions and conflict regarding care roles, boundaries, philosophies, and priorities. Collisions of any sort can generate tremendous energy, whether they involve atoms, automobiles, rain clouds, or people.

Collisions occur as the caregivers strive to meet their common goal of healthier or therapeutic communities. Caregivers wanted the best for the patient, parish, and community, but they often approached situations from different perspectives. In addition, sometimes patients wanted something different from the chaplain, parish nurse, and parish clergy. Their desires, wishes, and perceptions can also lead to collisions among caregivers.

For example, a parish nurse referred a young woman who had recently lost her husband to a grief support group held at one of the system hospitals. The woman was upset with God for taking her husband, and with her minister for not visiting her husband more frequently before his death. She was also upset with this clergy for not offering more help in her time of grief.

A parish nurse and hospital chaplain facilitated a grief group that she attended, but her anger at God and her minister prevented her from responding to the chaplain except with bitterness and hostility. Eventually, she stopped responding to the chaplain and responded to only the nurse. Her hostility toward the chaplain created tension and stress within the group and caused confusion and misunderstanding between the group facilitators.

The nurse facilitator approached the woman and encouraged her to discuss her reactions. The woman began sharing her experience and reason for her anger. The facilitator suggested that she discuss her anger with her parish nurse who could support her and make other appropriate referrals. The nurse facilitator encouraged the woman to share her story with the chaplain, but she refused. However, with the woman's permission, the nurse told the chaplain facilitator of the reasons for the hostility. Maintaining confidentiality and the woman's trust was of great importance.

This collision between the grieving woman and the hospital chaplain was directly related to past anger and hurt that contributed to continuing confusion and misunderstanding. Energy was generated by these collisions that, if left unresolved, could have led to isolation, and a negative and potentially detrimental situation for all involved. Communication between the nurse facilitator and the woman helped to make the situation less negative and hopefully led to more productive resolution in the future.

Complementarity

Connections among chaplains, parish nurses, and parish clergy can lead to productive complementarity in which those involved complement one another's practice skills, knowledge, and gifts to pursue the goal of healthier communities. Complementarity creates not only energy but also synergy that enhances the ideas and abilities of team members. Complementarity requires that team members be familiar with and have respect for the strengths of the others and be willing to utilize those strengths without regard to boundaries, ego, or personality characteristics. A case example demonstrating complementarity follows.

A woman was admitted with a poor prognosis to the intensive care unit of one of the system hospitals. Her only family member, a daughter, was informed of the news, and sought information regarding advanced directives. She was deeply religious and requested that the minister from her home congregation advise her on the procedure and on the "eternal consequences" of such an action. Her minister came immediately to the hospital and offered spiritual counsel. She became convinced that the advanced directive should be written and asked the minister to help with the procedure. He was unsure of the exact procedure and called the parish nurse for help. The parish nurse happened to work in that very hospital and knew the hospital chaplain. The nurse knew that chaplains were knowledgeable regarding advanced directives, and with the minister's approval, she called the chaplain.

The chaplain, parish nurse, and community clergy sat with the patient and her daughter while decisions were made and the forms were completed. Each team member offered support and encouragement to others in the room. At the close of the meeting, the patient asked for a prayer. Nobody knew who would say the prayer, and everyone waited for the others to speak.

For a brief moment it seemed as though a "turf war" could have ensued, but that did not happen. The community clergy suggested that everyone participate in the prayer who felt called to pray and asked if the chaplain, who was of a different denomination, would close the prayer. The result was a deep, rich, meaningful praise and petition during which everyone, including the patient, participated. After the prayer, the minister asked the chaplain and the parish nurse to continue checking on the mother and daughter. Later the minister thanked the parish nurse for bringing the chaplain to the situation, and expressed trust and a sense of friendship and kinship toward the chaplain.

CONCLUSION

As both health care institutions and congregations extend their efforts beyond their walls, hospital chaplains, parish nurses, and community clergy have opportunities to collaborate in pursuit of healthy communities. Hospital and congregational staff enter the community to cooperate in this shared mission. Each connection within and among the team has the potential for collisions or complementarity because although all three have a healing and wellness focus, each addresses the problem from a different perspective.

These collaborative community efforts create at least four positive outcomes. First, the natural bridge between congregation ministries and hospital services can strengthen the link between faith and health as congregations follow the clergy's direction toward healing and therapeutic communities. Second, greater support for these ministry programs is created as parishioners share their stories of successful participation and health care involvement with others. Third, more comprehensive care is provided as parishes and hospitals work together to coordinate and provide the highest level of holistic care. Fourth, chaplains, parish nurses, and community clergy have the opportunity to learn more about one another and their various roles within this healing mission.

Finally, each professional can utilize the skills and abilities of the others while discovering greater opportunities for collaboration. Collaborative efforts can include referral within one another's unique specialties, expert consultation across the fields of pastoral care and nursing, assistance with clinical improvement and community outreach programs, and development of educational programs geared toward staff, congregations, and communities. Through connection, with its potential for collision or complementarity, the community can embody the mission to help people be better, feel better, and carry suffering better.

REFERENCES

Evans, A. R. (1999). *Redeeming marketplace medicine: A theology of health care.* Cleveland, OH: Pilgrim Press.

Nelson, G. (1999). Pastoral reflections. In Solari-Twadell, P. A. and McDermott, M. A. (Eds.), *Parish nursing: Promoting whole person health within faith communities* (pp. 161-167). Thousand Oaks, CA: Sage Publications.

Schumann, R. R. (1999). Job description for the congregational nurse within the health ministry. *Ministry Directory* (pp. 12-13). Houston, TX: West University Church of Christ.

Chapter 16

Modeling the Wisdom of Journeying Together: Parish Nursing and Chaplaincy

Dan Magnus Geeding
Dorothea Honn

In the article "Weaving Spirituality into Organizational Life," Frederick Craigie (1998) described our concern and our vision. He states:

> A great deal of research and writing over the past two decades attest to the link between spirituality and health. The answer to the question "Does spirituality make a difference?" is clearly yes. It remains a challenge, however, even in organizations with germane mission statements and chaplaincy programs, to weave spirituality finely into the fabric of clinical care and organizational life. How can we operationalize spirituality and make it an integral part of the work and the workplace, of health care organizations? In other words, how can we think of spirituality not only as a clinical issue, but also as a vital organizational component of good clinical care? (p. 25)

To describe our experience, we begin with the minutes of our first pastoral care vision team meeting convened by the authors of this report who were designated as cochairs by hospital administration.

A version of this material was presented at the Thirteenth Annual Westberg Parish Nurse Symposium September 15-17, 1999, Itasca, Illinois.

The team appointed the vice president of inpatient services and the authors of this report as cochairs. The members decided that the goal of this multidisciplinary vision team was to develop a spiritual care delivery system for patients, their families, and care providers. The central question was "What does a spiritual care delivery system at the hospital look like to you?" The challenge for this task force was to define the vision, to share it with others, and then to find ways to realistically address spiritual needs. Incorporation of chaplaincy, parish nursing, clinical caregivers, and other local congregational/parish ministries were seen as working together to meet this goal. The vision team embraced the care delivery goal stated by the vice president that stressed the need for creating a caring, healthy work environment that responds to the spiritual needs of the patient, family, and employee. The vision team will meet approximately every six weeks to discuss the actions taken since the previous meeting. The team will address current issues and allow time for the shared visions, insights, and challenges from the group.

A key requirement for membership in the vision team was a passion for the development and implementation of spiritual care for patients, their families, and staff. The composition of the team included hospital administration, community pastors, chaplains, physicians, and an attorney who represents the community and the foundation of the hospital. Also represented were behavioral health, utilization review, medical oncology, women's health, social work, parish nursing, the fitness center, the retirement center, and hospice.

THE JOURNEY

The process of our journey is summarized into four categories: the ministry of relationships and modeling, implementation, evaluation, and our continuing challenge. A discussion of each follows.

THE MINISTRY OF RELATIONSHIPS AND MODELING

Where did this vision for increasing attention to spiritual needs come from? We reflected on the past and present. How is spirituality experienced and modeled within the institution? Who is encouraging additional attention to spirituality and why?

A foundation was laid in the past. It began in the community with the local ministerial association and their vision for effective pastoral care at the hospital. They established an emergency department volunteer chaplaincy and a local clergy continues to serve as the coordinator. They also influenced the hospital to secure a full-time paid chaplain, a program now in its second decade. The present chaplain reaps the benefits of the volunteer chaplains and the two full-time chaplains who preceded him. The current spiritual care delivery system is described in Figure 16.1. The vision and task of the present chaplain includes discovering creative ways to expand pastoral presence/spiritual care while being a one-person department. He expanded the focus and mission so that he can respond more adequately to the needs of patients, family members, hospital staff, and physicians. When he relates to staff as spiritual caregivers themselves, they increasingly identify and own the influence of their own spirituality, expanding their attention to spiritual care.

Approximately four years ago, a parish nursing program began at the same time as a new chaplain arrived. The parish nurses worked with staff nurses in the clinical setting, modeling spiritual presence. This encouraged staff nurses to explore and enhance the spiritual side of being a caregiver. The parish nurses have also established relationships with local congregations and social service agencies as portrayed in Figure 16.2.

Another foundation for the current interest in spiritual care came from an incident within the institution in which a family's emotional and spiritual needs were not met after a sudden death. The situation was complicated by incorrect family data provided to staff members in several departments. The chaplain and parish nurse were requested to address and correct the issue. Hmm! The challenge! Given the vision process described previously, we realized that this was an invitation to do more than provide a bandage. Administration gave permission for the development of a vision team. Its goal was to build a team approach with input from the community as the chaplain and parish nurse joined with clergy and community churches.

FIGURE 16.1. Spiritual Care Delivery System

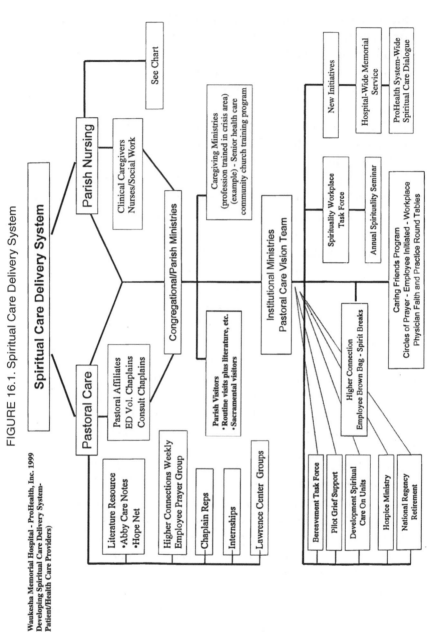

Waukesha Memorial Hospital - ProHealth, Inc. 1999
Developing Spiritual Care Delivery System-
Patient/Health Care Providers)

FIGURE 16.2. Relationships Among Parish Nurses, Congregations, and Service Agencies

For the Benefit of Our Community

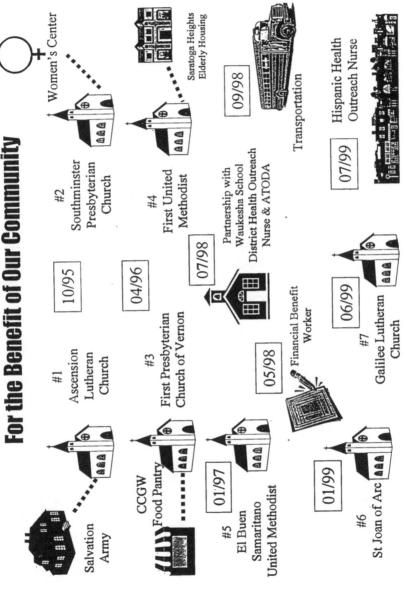

Women's Center

Saratoga Heights
Elderly Housing

09/98

Transportation

Hispanic Health
Outreach Nurse

07/99

#2
Southminster
Presbyterian
Church

#4
First United
Methodist

Partnership with
Waukesha School
District Health Outreach
Nurse & ATODA

07/98

10/95

04/96

#1
Ascension
Lutheran
Church

#3
First Presbyterian
Church of Vernon

Financial Benefit
Worker

05/98

#7
Galilee Lutheran
Church

06/99

Salvation
Army

CCGW
Food Pantry

01/97

01/99

#5
El Buen
Samaritano
United Methodist

#6
St Joan of Arc

The mission of the vision team was also validated and encouraged by three patients rights standards put in place January 1, 1997, by the Joint Commission for the Accreditation of Healthcare Organizations. These standards remain in their quarterly updates:

> Standard RI.1.2: Patients are involved in all aspects of their care. Patients' psychological, spiritual, and cultural values affect how they respond to their care. The hospital allows patients and their families to express their spiritual beliefs and cultural practices, as long as these do not harm others or interfere with treatment.
>
> Standard RI.1.2.7: The hospital addresses care at the end of life. Dying patients have unique needs for respectful, responsive care. All hospital staff is sensitized to the needs of patients at the end of life. . . . The hospital's framework for addressing issues related to care at the end of life provides for respecting the patient's values, religion, and philosophy, . . . responding to the . . . concerns of the patient and the family.
>
> Standard RI.1.3.5: The hospital demonstrates respect for the following patient needs: confidentiality, privacy, security, resolution of complaints, pastoral care and other spiritual services. . . . Hospitals respect and provide for each patient's right to pastoral counseling. It is recognized that services for patients' spiritual needs may be provided by clergy or certified chaplains as well as individuals who are not ordained or certified. Therefore services are provided or available in a variety of ways. (pp. RI.13-16)

What was our starting point? Yes, we had an incident—but it was far more than that. The institution was blessed with staff members who had the vision for an improved spiritual care delivery system and a vice president who was passionately involved with and supportive of both chaplaincy and parish nursing. We had a sense that God was leading us.

As cofacilitators, what did we hear at our first vision team meeting when we asked, "What does a spiritual care delivery system at the hospital look like to you?" The various comments of the representatives identified the task of converting dreams into reality. A summary statement of the vision team articulated the dream:

An enthusiastic group of visionaries met with an appreciation and sense of encouragement from the hospital to recognize and respond to spiritual needs of patients, families, and staff. We named and put into writing what spiritual emphases were already in place. Persons from various work areas shared the goal of increasing spirituality development. We talked about not only education and training of clinical caregivers to respond to the needs of patients, families, and staff but the importance of modeling spirituality in relationships. How do we go about accomplishing this? How do we give each other permission? We named the importance of assessment skills in triaging needs, knowing our limitations, and the importance of timing for appropriate referral.

Comments from this first vision meeting also produced specific concerns. They were as follows:

- Clinical caregivers need grief counseling/guidance and training.
- How can we give permission to talk about spiritual concerns?
- The hospital needs to recognize and encourage staff members to respond to spiritual needs.
- How do we help patients/staff express their spirituality with or without religion?
- We need to know whether the immediate staff person can respond to the needs in the patient situation or whether referral to chaplaincy is necessary.
- We need to know limitations.
- It is important to communicate to the community what the hospital is doing to respond to spiritual needs.
- We need to meet the needs of home care/assisted living/short- and long-term care and family living apart from their loved ones.
- What is our focus? Where on the continuum do we give support?
- Where do we touch that patient's life?
- Critical care nurses need to tell us ways in which they would like to see spiritual concerns in the intensive care units addressed.
- We need to improve care to families experiencing the death of loved one.

In this meeting, we also observed and heard individual expressions of pain in regard to structuring new roles and a lack of shared knowledge about present roles in the institution.

We were developing a ministry of relationships. We were listening to one another and sharing what we heard and perceived. We were developing an awareness of who we were and what we offered, encouraging the process of identifying perceived and experienced needs.

Two and a half years into the development of our spiritual care delivery system we discovered Richard W. Smith's (1998) article "Attending to the Spirit." His statements provided additional validation of our journey.

> Servant leadership is about deep identity at three levels: personal, relational, and institutional. It asks the questions: who am I? who are we and why do we choose to have the relationships we do? . . . [L]eadership is a way of being, more concerned with relationships and connections than role definition.
>
> . . . [A]s servant leaders evolve, they co-create community, shaping the environment for themselves and others. Servant leaders are listeners.
>
> . . . [S]ervant leaders use power ethically, persuade rather than manipulate or coerce, and accept the responsibility of accountability in all three spheres: personal, relational and institutional. (pp. 30-31)

As a further starting point, why would a parish nurse and a chaplain join together to facilitate the development of a spiritual care delivery system? Yes, we were asked to by the hospital administration! We also began to converse and reflect on our roles within the institution and the community—the wisdom of a ministry of relationships, the values of being a team, and the value of what can happen. A ministry of modeling was being experienced and expressed.

We also found it important to identify specific gifts, skills, and talents that the chaplain and parish nurse brought to this ministry. Those of the chaplain included these:

- Providing a constant presence in the institution
- Facilitating communication, delegation, and referral

- Functioning as a consultant and resource person for parish nurses
- Identifying the value of theological reflection and exploring different faith traditions
- Facilitating communication and a continual sounding board for pastors and parish nurses
- Serving as a mediator/presence in conflict resolution
- Offering experience and insight from clinical and pastoral settings

Parish nurses have bidimensional roles. Those in the congregation are as follows:

- Addressing congregational wellness
- Providing health education
- Functioning as health counselor
- Providing advocacy
- Referral

Those in the hospital setting include these:

- Providing liaisons between the parish nursing program and chaplaincy
- Facilitating staff awareness of spiritual care initiatives and reinforcing them
- Serving as a clinical consultant in the identification of spiritual needs (This process helps inform and provides education regarding "presence" ministry and the need for chaplaincy care.)
- Providing understanding and promoting appreciation regarding the roots and function of chaplaincy/pastoral-spiritual care

In our own way we were experiencing the reality conveyed by William Bazan and Daniel Dwyer (1998) in their article "Assessing Spirituality." They wrote:

> Organizations do not need to make people spiritual; spirituality does not develop from the outside. Even though everyone is born with a spiritual nature—a center of personal power—one's spiritual capacity is often hidden, rather like a financial treasure

growing in a savings account one does not know one has. Once they discover that they have this treasure, they can access its energy and power. (p. 24)

IMPLEMENTATION OF VISION INTO REALITY

Implementation included an understanding of what is true, right, and lasting. The importance of scriptural passages became evident in the development of clinical spiritual care.

> I alone know the plans I have for you, plans to bring you prosperity and not disaster, plans to bring about the future you hope for. Then you will call to me. You will come and pray to me, and I will answer you. You will seek me, and you will find me because you seek me with all your heart. (Jeremiah 29:11-13)

> Who then is Paul, and who is Apollos, but ministers by whom you believed, as the Lord gave to each one? I have planted, Apollos watered, but God gave the increase. So then neither he who plans is anything, nor he who waters, but God who gives the increase. (I Corinthians 3:5-7, NKJV)

> Fix your thoughts on what is true and good and right. Think about things that are pure and lovely, and dwell on the fine, good things in others. Think about all you can praise God for and be glad about. Keep putting into practice all you learned from me and saw me doing, and the God of peace will be with you. (Philippians 3:8-9, TLB)

It was important for us to understand our institutions' organizational system and framework. We saw the importance of solid documentation in policies and procedures regarding the process of meeting spiritual needs. The wisdom of living creatively, and somewhat dangerously, within our boundaries also existed. We started with the present situation, moving forward from that point.

The value of the interprofessional team and the importance of community evolved as key components of this ministry. Our efforts were validated by employee responses. In turn, we identified employees who were gifted with spiritual administrative leadership. This empowered the process of implementing spiritual care in our workplace and facilitating ownership of spiritual care by the caregivers themselves.

EVALUATING OUR JOURNEY

The ministry of evaluation discovered areas that required improvement. We increasingly value the role of the multidisciplinary team process in spiritual care delivery. It requires that "turf wars" cease and that individuals be open to the value of the different roles of the interdisciplinary members and what each offers. The provision of spiritual care has no room for "Lone Rangers."

Someone once said that people could be so "heavenly minded" that they were of no "earthly good." We believe three things are crucial in keeping us grounded:

- Empowerment and endorsement of administration and institutional leadership
- Creativity in presenting new spiritual care initiatives, such as these:
    Employee brown bag lunches—spirit break
    Spirituality in the workplace—annual conference
    Bereavement task force and pilot bereavement support group
- Employee ownership of spirituality in the workplace (In our setting, this consists of the employee caring friends program, the high connections employee prayer group, employee-initiated circles of prayer for crisis care and support for one another, and the physician faith and practice roundtables).

OUR CONTINUED CHALLENGE

Our challenge today is to grow, evaluate, and take initiatives in discovering how to continually facilitate positive spiritual changes. We continue to believe that our experiences affirm a special truth expressed by Joseph Gillespie (1998): "we can allow the surprise of life to happen, allow spirituality to inform us rather than conform us" (p. 33). Our ever-expanding team reflected in Figure 16.1 is modeling the message that spirituality needs to be inclusive, is learning some commonality in defining itself, and is experiencing the joy of living it! In the continued development of spiritual care delivery, the emphasis of Bazan and Dwyer (1998) continue to speak to us: "Relational power and presence represent the capacity to: nurture and sustain personal and professional relationships. Individuals experience this presence as a process of giving and receiving, of influencing and being influenced. It is a two-way street" (p. 22).

REFERENCES

Bazan, William J. and Dwyer, Daniel (1998). Assessing spirituality. *Health Progress,* March/April, 20-24.

Craigie, Frederick C., Jr. (1998). Weaving spirituality into organizational life. *Health Progress,* March/April, 25-28.

Gillespie, Joseph (1998). Everyday spirituality can help healthcare professionals sustain their passion. *Health Progress,* July/August, 32-33.

Joint Commission for the Accreditation of Healthcare Institutions (1997). Comprehensive accreditation manual for hospitals: Standards: Patient rights and organizational ethics. Oakbrook Terrace, IL: Joint Commission on Accreditation of Healthcare Organizations, RI-4-RI16.

Smith, Richard W. (1998). Attending to the spirit. *Health Progress,* July/August, 30-31.

SECTION VI:
RELATIONSHIPS TO
HEALTH CARE INSTITUTIONS

Chapter 17

The Role of the Health Care Institution in Pastor and Parish Nurse Team Building

Linda L. Pape

Parish nursing is increasingly well known within the nursing profession, faith communities, and health care institutions. Health care institutions have been major initiators of parish nurse networks throughout parish nursing's fifteen-year history. Most of these institutions comprise faith-based hospitals, nursing homes, or other local health care providers. Without this institutional support, parish nursing would not have the stature it enjoys today. I believe that the contributions of health care institutions need to continue for some time to bring stability and definition to the practice of parish nursing.

Those who have shaped parish nursing practice include the International Parish Nurse Resource Center,[1] the Health Ministries Association (HMA),[2] faith-based health care institutions, and the parish nurses themselves. Churches and other faith communities also have recently fanned the flames of parish nursing services. Only within the last couple of years have organizations such as the American Nurses Association (ANA) or the various state associations taken a role in parish nursing growth and activity. Many academic nursing programs recently joined these initiatives, providing basic and advanced courses for parish nurses.

Some health care institutions provide a full-time or part-time coordinator to support and educate parish nurses, helping them define their role and function within faith communities. It is from such a coordinator role that I share my observations and comments here. In this chapter I will

- briefly explain how a health care institution supports parish nurse programs within our community;

- share my observations of parish nurse, pastoral staff, and congregational working relationships and factors that may influence them; and
- outline ways that health care institutions may positively influence individual parish nurse programs.

My particular view of each situation is from outside the congregation and is influenced by what parish nurses report to me. I see those relationships which seem to work well, those which need improvement, and those which appear to be in serious difficulty. I witness the impact of success or failure on parish nurses and health ministry programs.

THE INSTITUTION'S SUPPORT
OF THE VOLUNTEER PARISH NURSE PROGRAM

Grant/Riverside Methodist Hospitals, a large health system in central Ohio, has sponsored a volunteer parish nurse program since 1992. It offers support to congregations not only from the church partnerships department but also from many parts of our health care system. Examples include clinical pastoral education (CPE) offered to parish nurses from the pastoral care department and the grief training workshops offered by the hospice program. The institution offers heart health educational programs to African-American congregations through a program titled "Doin' the Right Healthy Thing." Most congregations, however, interface with our organization's parish nurse and health ministry programs through the church partnership department, where two coordinators serve as liaisons to the communities of faith, one for parish nursing and one for general health ministry.

As parish nurse coordinator of this volunteer model, I observe how new parish nurses define their role within the faith community. My position of institutional coordinator has many roles: encourager, facilitator, educator, and supporter of parish nurses who work in their local congregations in a paid or nonpaid position.

Functions of the coordinator role include the following:

- Providing consultation to congregations as they develop and maintain parish nurse programs
- Organizing orientation and educational workshops

- Providing support groups for parish nurses and liaisons from the congregations
- Assisting in measuring the program's impact on the churches and the broader community
- Serving as a window to the institution's assets that can benefit the congregation and community
- Serving as personal advisor and support to the practicing parish nurse

From this personal advisor and support role I gain most of my insights into the working relationships between nurses, clergy, and congregations.

As coordinator of a volunteer parish nurse program, my interactions are most often with the nurses who serve as liaisons between the congregation and our institution's church partnerships department. As a parish nurse coordinator, I work with approximately thirty-six parish nurses in as many faith communities. Admittedly my time is limited, and I spend quality one-on-one time with each nurse approximately twice per year. Most of our conversations are at meetings, workshops, or by phone as the need arises.

Some parish nurses, both paid and volunteer, spend forty or more hours per week in their role. Others spend only a few hours per month. Minimum requirements are not made for participation in our network and only eternity will measure the true fruit of their labor. Some nurses work mostly alone and are considered "the parish nurse" of the church while others work within large health ministry teams composed of professionals and laity, each filling a different role. In the latter example, however, I always work with a liaison who represents the church.

A CONTINUUM OF PARISH NURSE
AND PASTORAL STAFF RELATIONSHIPS

I categorize the parish nurse and pastoral staff relationships into three groups: (1) synergistic and collaborative, (2) limited partnering, and (3) antagonistic and nonsupportive. Obviously this oversimplifies the working relationships represented in our network, but it provides a means for discussion and analysis. Most relationships fall within the limited-partnering area and they receive the most discussion here.

The Synergistic and Collaborative Relationship

First, I define how I use the term "synergistic." This occurs in those "best marriages" in which the sum of the two people adds up to more than the two individuals. The communication levels are good, they strive for the same goals, they respect each other, and what they produce together is good. As with good marriages, the nurse and clergy work very well together in situations associated with individual parishioners in crises. Both the clergy and nurse move in and out of situations and they truly complement each other. They may also make team visits to utilize their various gifts.

Another very positive working relationship that I observe in parish nursing practice is "true collaboration," which may or may not involve true "synergy." Clergy and nurse may work side by side in the congregation, greatly respect each other's efforts, but for the most part work separately. They might describe themselves as having their own distinctive roles.

Whether synergistic or collaborative, these parish nurses display at least five similar characteristics.

- They are mature in their decision-making process and most often have held leading church roles long before beginning their nursing practice. In our volunteer model, nearly all the parish nurses come from the churches they now serve. This differs from many paid models elsewhere. Two of the nurses whom I identify with this category were nurse leaders in the church prior to the advent of parish nursing.
- Spiritual maturity is also evident. This strengthens the nurse's ability to establish increasing peership with the clergy.
- Each has an in-depth knowledge of parish nursing and has prepared for the task both educationally and personally.
- Parish nurses in this category have a strong self-identity and are good team players.
- Each of these nurses truly loves the congregation and has a spiritual commitment to service.

All of the parish nurses in this first group have worked out a role definition with their pastoral partners. They meet regularly with the clergy and are included in staff meetings, whether they are in paid or nonpaid positions. Often this "being part of staff meetings" develops over time or during the "testing" of this new position.

The Limited-Partnering Parish Nurse and Pastor Relationship

Other coordinators in the field as well as myself believe that the limited-partnering relationship is the most frequent. Although I believe the synergistic and collaborative relationship is the ideal, a limited partnership can be very productive. It can progress to the synergistic or collaborative level with mutual commitment to learn from each other.

Several factors significantly influence the partnership of parish nurses, pastoral staff, and congregation. Parish nurse factors will be discussed first, followed by pastoral staff and congregational factors.

Parish Nurse Factors

Many factors may prevent the parish nurse from becoming more involved, including time limitations, the need for income/reimbursement, and a lack of commitment. In addition, the education and skills of the nurse may not sufficiently match the position or the needs of the congregation. These limiting factors may be legitimate and unavoidable; others can sometimes be overcome with proper planning and evaluation. A discussion of each concern follows.

Time Commitment. The nurse may be semiretired or spend time away from the congregation part of the year. Many have recently left the full-time workforce and do not want to dedicate large blocks of time to a volunteer position. Many more do not find others to share the workload, may experience symptoms of burnout, and leave the role. With strong committee oversight this model may provide good service, but the program does not contain the same sense of identity or visibility that is present during full integration. These nurses are rarely incorporated into the church staff.

Rewards and Reimbursement Issues. Commitment and involvement may also be greatly affected if the parish nurse does not receive some form of reimbursement. Even a small budget with some paid expenses has a big impact on commitment because it gives stature and recognition to the program and possible assurance of its continuation. Many parish nurses give as much or greater time than the minister of music or religious education director. Identification of and value attributed to the position by the pastoral staff and parishioners are also closely associated to this budget factor.

Do I feel that volunteer parish nurse programs are inferior to paid programs? No, but I do believe the longevity and durability of parish nursing rests with reimbursement and recognition of services. Too many volunteer parish nurses feel unappreciated and taken for granted after a period of time. They may lose interest and even leave practice. Those parish nurses who do not wish to be paid even when it is offered should report the gift value of the nonpaid staff position and record the equivalent cash value of their work in order to increase recognition of the program.

Beyond the reimbursement issue is the recognition that the clergy and congregation give to the program. Often this is just a note or special thank-you that recognizes the parish nurse in some unique way. Volunteer recognition reaps bountiful rewards within the congregation.

The "Volunteer Time" Mentality versus the "Professional Parish Nurse" Mentality. For many, the practice of parish nursing on a volunteer basis is seen as having less commitment. Parish nurses may say, "I want to give of my time and not do all that paperwork anymore." They want to volunteer but do not want to be burdened by many demands. When parish nurses do not articulate their level of involvement clearly, congregational leadership can find it very confusing. To avoid this confusion, parish nurses need to write realistic descriptions of their expectations, including goals and objectives, for their colleagues to examine before beginning service. If the commitment changes, this should also be described in writing.

A "volunteer parish nurse" must still abide by the *Scope and Standards of Parish Nursing Practice* (HMA/ANA,1998). One nurse recently stated, "All I want to do is take blood pressures." When such limited intentions are present, I recommend that she not call herself a parish nurse. This nurse might be wiser to say, "I wish to support the health ministry of the congregation by taking blood pressures on a monthly basis." When individuals proclaim themselves "parish nurses" for the congregation, it conveys a larger commitment than doing one task on an irregular schedule. This clarification would also avoid unrealistic expectations of the pastoral staff and congregation.

Sadly, many parish nurses do not create a clear understanding concerning the services that they wish to deliver. Thus, the "business" of parish nursing never takes hold and disappointed clergy may not support such efforts in the future.

Education, Preparation, and Skills of the Parish Nurse. Formal education, preparation, and communication skills all contribute to defining relationships. Although standards of parish nursing are recognized, a standardized preparation for practice does not yet exist. All registered nurses can presently call themselves parish nurses without being challenged. They can receive orientation or education in many ways, including self-study preparation or formal college courses in parish nursing. How clergy and church committees view parish nurses and their ability to practice in the church can be influenced by recognition of proper preparation. Most clergy receive formal seminary education to prepare themselves for the pastoral role and demonstrate readiness for pastoral practice through some form of endorsement or ordination process. It is understandable that they might question the ability of a paid or nonpaid staff who has not obtained qualified preparation or demonstrated readiness for practice.

Communication skills are the number one prerequisite for building parish nurse relationships. In our summer parish nursing course offered at a local college, we emphasize systems theory and its application to the church environment. Nurses who understand denominational structures and relationships within the local church will have a head start in integrating their ministry.

Clergy and Congregational Leadership Factors

Congregational factors influencing a lack of support include these:

- Contradictory understandings and differing philosophies
- Inability to share responsibilities
- Ego and personality conflicts

A description of each factor follows.

Understanding Each Other's Unique Professional Perspective and Language. The underlying philosophy of parish nursing is central to its success. Its foundation is the assumption that ministry to body, mind, and spirit involves the whole person. The pastoral staff members or congregational leaders may not grasp its meaning or understand what is involved in implementing such a perspective within the congregation. Communicating this perspective along with doctrinal explanations is essential for those providing services. Frequently, neither the clergy nor the nurse spends sufficient time building this foundation for service.

Frankly, if a clergy does not believe in health ministry within the church, it most often will not happen. And if there is half-hearted support by either party, the program will be negatively affected in some way. One equation must always be present: a clergy and a nurse must be truly committed and supportive of each other.

Inability to Share Responsibilities. Parish nursing combines spiritual care with nursing skills in unique ways. Some clergy, however, may be threatened by another (nonpastor) filling a spiritual ministry role and this can relegate the parish nurse to a medical model of practice within the congregation. In some parishes, conflict is focused in the relationship between the parish nurse and the "retired" visitation pastor of the congregation.

Conversely, some parish nurses prefer the medical model of care and many need assistance in learning how to provide spiritual care. They often share functions with some other professions. For example, a good parish nurse often utilizes skills claimed by social workers. Some parish nurses have completed seminary courses. This is very congruent with the practice of parish nursing because it combines recognized nursing skills with spiritual ministry. Many parish nurses along with ministers or other pastoral staff frequently say, "I am called to ministry."

Egos and Conflicts. Both clergy and parish nurses can have strong egos, and how they construct their relationship is central to success or failure. Most parish nurses have dwelt with many strong-willed doctors in previous nursing positions. The negotiation skills and finesse they have developed over the years are also necessary within the church structure. Building this relationship with clergy can be difficult although the clergy must not be singled out in this regard. I have, however, seen clergy use their power to enhance their egos. I have observed several excellent parish nurses leave practice because they did not have the necessary skills to deal with the egos of the pastoral staff. Conversely, the parish nurses were too inflexible, unable to compromise or negotiate the congregational system. To have a good working relationship with the clergy, the nurse must be competent and politically astute.

In summary, the limited-partnering practice, even with its drawbacks, still provides multiple assets for the congregation and the field of parish nursing. Addressing these drawbacks will promote movement into the synergistic/collaborative relationship.

Antagonistic and Nonsupportive Parish Nurse-Pastor Relationship

Antagonistic and nonsupportive relationships are opposite the synergistic/collaborative style. They occur in noncompatible relationships between the parish nurse, pastoral staff members, and the congregation.

Noncompatibility

I have observed a few situations in this category. In two instances, persons just wanted to be parish nurses and the clergy placated the nurses or a strong faction within the congregation by letting it happen. Those outside the situations could clearly see that the clergy were not backing the programs. In other cases, programs begun under clergy who provided good support encountered new leadership that demonstrated little interest so the programs were not maintained. With congregations that change pastors regularly, I have observed a strong program remain by simply waiting out the nonsupportive leadership.

I encourage congregations that put a high priority on health ministry to showcase the program when searching for a new clergy. Some congregations have educated prospective candidates by making videos that include the parish nurse program. When the new pastoral staff arrives, the parish nurse and health committee must educate the staff regarding all aspects of the program.

Not the Right Time

Even though church leadership may view the parish nurse program as valuable, it may be the wrong time. A health ministry may need to be delayed when other issues are taking all the energy and resources.

Examples include churches that are "between pastors" and when a new building campaign is in progress. Only a couple of congregations with which I have worked started a program without a senior clergy on-site.

I have observed a couple of persistent parish nurses leave one church and move to another situation where they could then fulfill their desire to serve. One parish nurse left her own church to go to a paid position in another denomination, which worked well.

Parish nurses may fall out of favor if they are not meeting the expectations of the pastoral leadership or the committee's desires for the program. This again supports the need for good communication, clear goal setting, and periodic review of program effectiveness.

As parish nurse coordinator, I am learning to boldly verbalize non-compatibility signs that I observe. I admit to not wanting to bring bad tidings or crush hopes of those truly desiring to be involved in health ministry within their congregation, but I have urged some "would be" parish nurses to consider a different congregation for practice.

THE INSTITUTION'S AND PARISH NURSE COORDINATOR'S ROLES IN SUPPORTING PROGRAMS AND GOOD WORKING RELATIONSHIPS

Parameters of the Relationship Between Congregation and Health Care Institution

Many health care institutions are willing to work with congregations in an ongoing relationship when it is mutually beneficial and affects the health and welfare of the community. Both bring gifts and abilities that can contribute to a positive impact on promoting health and preventing illness. In addition, faith-based health care institutions often share common values with communities of faith.

Institutions support parish nursing in various ways. The first model outlined in *The Parish Nurse* (Westberg and Westberg McNamara, 1990) provides direct oversight for the parish nurse. Some models provide various monetary and in-kind supports to congregational parish nurse programs. Ours is a "volunteer model" with the congregation assuming ownership and primary support for its program. The three primary benefits provided to the congregation by our institution are resources, supervision, and support. A discussion of each follows.

Resources

Congregations often approach health care institutions for resources, perhaps to support a health fair or speaker, or to initiate a parish nurse program. Our church partnerships program has grown at the same time as our health care system has dwelt with reduced funding and several mergers. We have offered the following specific resources rather than salaries or other monetary gifts to congregations who are beginning programs.

Hospital-Based Coordinator and Educational Resources

This health care institution makes a large commitment by providing two paid coordinators to educate, support, and provide consultation to congregations. This provides free, high-quality education from many departments, including pastoral care, employee education, social services, hospice, and many specialty services such as heart, mental health, and cancer care. The hospital library provides current educational materials and videos for partnership congregations. CPE courses are available through the pastoral care department. We provide cardiopulmonary resuscitation (CPR) training and specialty education for parish nurses, enabling them to remain current in practice. We partner with a local college to provide parish nurse courses for master's, bachelor's, and continuing education needs. Ours is not an exclusive relationship; congregations are encouraged to utilize all resources available within the community.

Monetary Support versus Shared Resources and Gifts

Most congregations want to own and control their program, looking to the health care organization for resources and support. Several clergy and health committees clearly state that they do not want more institutional ownership. I believe this does not threaten the partnering relationship but instead serves as its strength.

Although health care institutions are valuable resources, many are being forced to withdraw financial support for parish nurse programs in congregations. For this reason I believe that the volunteer institutional model is a viable one and parish nurse programs are more likely to remain if institutional maintenance is withdrawn. In time, I believe congregations of all denominations will need to provide more monetary support for parish nurse programs.

What then does our institution want in return for its resources? It wants measured productivity and outcomes of the parish nurse programs. All parish nurses complete a quarterly report that describes the differences they make. These reports support our organization's congregational partnerships, but they also provide the parish nurse, health committee, and congregation validation for continuing and often enhancing the program. Several of the parish nurses in our network can attribute their paid status to the measured outcomes they reported.

Supervision of the Parish Nurse Program

Supervision is probably the major reason congregations involve an institution in the development and oversight of a parish nurse program. Health care institutions have nurses who understand nursing practice and coordinators who hopefully combine the technical knowledge and skills with interest in spiritual ministry. The quality of help offered by institutions probably depends on the individual coordinator. I believe high standards need to be set for this individual as she or he indeed can make or break programs affiliated with the institution.

Some institutions take a very active oversight role, monitoring day-to-day activities. Our institution takes an advisory role, leaving most of the oversight obligations to the congregation. We educate and counsel regarding practice matters and spell out specific requirements, but administration of the daily practice is handled within the congregational structure. Some view this stance positively while others have concerns. Most of our partnership congregations want control over the program within the church; others feel unprepared because of liability concerns. Having a reputable institutional parish nurse partnership does assist the congregation in providing a safer and more stable program.

General Support for the Parish Nurse Program

The Parish Nurse and Health Ministry Forum

From the beginning, institutional support groups sponsored by the health care institution provided forums for parish nurses to meet one another and to discuss mutual concerns. These monthly meetings are valued by parish nurses and provide reassurance that they are not alone. Ongoing education, community service orientation, oversight, and spiritual sharing create strong bonds in our monthly parish nurse and health ministry forum. The committees of the forum decide direction and content. Relationship topics are included and we have had teams of parish nurses and pastoral staff members present to this group.

The forum's mentoring committee is beginning new plans to strengthen leadership for new parish nurses and provide stronger support for role development. We have even discussed having parish nurse/pastoral teams as mentors for the network.

Consulting Services

Beyond free consultations available through our church partnerships department, we hold regular meetings with partnership congregations. These meetings often include the clergy, the parish nurse, and the coordinator who together review the status of the program and its plans. Feedback concerning congregational activity is shared, and clergy who support the program utilize this time to call attention to the contributions of the parish nurse. Infrequently meetings include discussions about working relationships or role definition issues.

The coordinator may also provide consultation services outside the local area. Such consultations aim to prevent problems in new or existing programs.

Clergy from our partnership churches participate in focus groups that fill an advisory and consultation role for our program. From time to time we ask for their help in dealing with community health issues. Several clergy have also collaborated in our effort to obtain health-related grants for community projects.

We celebrate the achievements of the parish nurses and invite their clergy and committees to contribute comments for special recognition. It still remains a challenge to consistently get good attendance on these occasions.

Counselor and Confidant(e)

By far the largest role I play is that of confidante, counselor, and friend to the individual parish nurse. Often I drop what I am doing to meet with a nurse who is concerned about a situation with a parishioner or a working relationship. Most often the nurse simply needs someone to listen regarding a stressful relationship or event. Nurses often feel very alone in their role and need a great deal of support to continue. This sharing is treated with respect and confidentiality.

SUMMARY

In this program, both the health system and the congregational partners give and receive. No money changes hands but the benefits for both are significant. I am sure that many of our congregations would not be involved with parish nursing programs without the organization's support. The health system also benefits by building relationships with the faith community. Besides showing evidence of our parish nurse program, we are able to display concrete health promotion and illness prevention outcomes represented by the work of many congregations. As a health care institution we stand ready to provide support, education, and resources and hopefully fan the flames of what the community of faith can accomplish.

NOTES

1. The International Parish Nurse Resource Center, 205 W. Touhy, Suite 104, Park Ridge, IL 60068. Director: Phyllis Ann Solari-Twadell. Phone: 1-800-556-5368.

2. Health Ministries Association, P.O. Box 7178, Atlanta, GA 30357-0187. Phone: 1-800-280-9919.

REFERENCES

Health Ministries Association/American Nurses Association 1998. *Scope and Standards of Parish Nursing Practice.* Washington, DC: American Nurses Publishing.

Solari-Twadell, P. A. and McDermott, M. A. (1999). *Parish nursing: Promoting whole person health within faith communities.* Thousand Oaks, CA: Sage Publications, pp. 17-20.

Westberg, G. and Westberg McNamara, J. 1990. *The parish nurse: Providing a minister of health for your congregation.* Minneapolis, MN: Augsburg Fortress.

Chapter 18

Theoretical Models of Parish Nursing, Chaplains, and Community Clergy Interdisciplinary Relationships

Sybil D. Smith

Parish nurses, chaplains, and community clergy increasingly recognize the need to collaborate. The marketplace values driving the American health delivery system generate problems requiring interdisciplinary and collaborative solutions. In addition, research foundations and other funding sources increasingly value health care delivered in the community by interdisciplinary and collaborative efforts. This interdisciplinary and collaborative approach, however, is problematic; years of documentation describe its difficulties and tensions (Auerswald, 1968; Davis, 1997; McDaniel and Campbell, 1997; Panel Discussion, 1997; Schein, 1972). This chapter offers a theoretical lens through which to view the underlying philosophies at the heart of parish nursing programs and explores one structured, systematic way to think about interdisciplinary collaboration.

In this discussion, parish nurses are registered professionals who promote health and wholeness as members of the ministry staff in a faith community (Health Ministries Association and American Nurses Association [HMA and ANA], 1998). Each state defines parish nursing practice by the Nurse Practice Act and the *Scope and Standards of Parish Nursing Practice* (HMA and ANA, 1998). Chaplains are ordained or commissioned clergy who provide pastoral care services within a health care organization. Their ministry focuses on the care of the soul and is defined by the employing organization. A community clergy is a professional who provides administration, celebration, proclamation, and teaching to a congregation or parish.

UNDERLYING PHILOSOPHY

Parish nurse programs are saturated with Westberg's approach and they often appear pragmatic and difficult to evaluate (Westberg, 1990). This chapter creates an interdisciplinary and systematic classification of these programs. The task of an interdisciplinary group becomes more transparent when its aims and purposes are defined. Three theoretical models are described in an effort to establish some interdisciplinary common ground. These include the mission/ministry model, the marketplace model, and the access model (Smith, 1999, 2000a, 2000b). The purpose is to develop interdisciplinary perspective by clarifying the confusion regarding program evaluation and outcome measurement (Buckhart, 1997; Magilvy and Brown, 1997; McClosky, 1997; Rydholm, 1997). Four components of each model are discussed: the parish nurse, the authority of the parish nurse program, the substance of the parish nurse program, and the interface between the parish nurse, the chaplain, and the parish clergy.

MISSION/MINISTRY MODEL

The Parish Nurse

In the mission/ministry model, the parish nurse is either unpaid or paid staff on the ministry team of the congregation. The parish nurse spiritually discerns a call to congregational care ministry, serves as a steward of the faith, and ministers within a home congregation from a whole-person health perspective. The parish nurse is a professional but is considered a lay minister unless commissioned by a religious body.

Authority for the Parish Nurse Program

In this model, the nurse finds purpose and meaning in rendering ministry on behalf of the faith. Mission answers the "why" and ministry answers the "what" (Miller, 1997). Authority comes from being called by God to ministry and being installed by the parish to perform that ministry, although denominations differ as to the nature and extent of that authority, as evident when the functions of laity and clergy are compared. The parish nurse serves the parish at the pleasure of the clergy, board, or organizational structure, and for the purposes defined by the ministry plan of the parish. The clergy, in turn, are bound by ecclesiastical responsibility for the parish. Clergy often do not control the ministry of the parish but their leadership role makes them a credible gatekeeper. Objectives of the parish nurse ministry are directed by the ministry goals of the parish through designated processes and structures. Therefore, entering into the ministry of the parish is dependent on whether parish authorities desire such a ministry and what the nurse can bring to it.

Substance of the Parish Nurse Program

Faith formation is a core purpose of the parish and the context within which to understand the integration of faith and health (Smith, 1999). The journey of faith moves toward health, healing, and wholeness as it embraces the ministry of reconciliation and love (Bakken, 1987; Beckmen, 1995; Miller, 1997). Wholeness is considered to be *shalom* wholeness, or being at peace and harmony in all relationships. Thus, nurses practicing in this model find personal meaning and purpose in the ministry of congregational care, and in that role, they are one with the congregation they serve. In Christian solidarity and parishioner-focused care, the nurses both find and share the healing ministry of Jesus in the congregation where God's word is proclaimed, sins are confessed and forgiven, and the sacraments are practiced in fellowship with Christians. Congregations promote health by nurturing spiritual values and by sponsoring health-related programs (Miller, 1997). The focus is not on the role of the nurse but on the needs of the persons served by the ministry (Smith, 2000a).

Interface with Health Care Chaplains

The parish nurse may seek services of chaplains in meeting the needs of the congregation. For instance, the nurse may seek assistance with certain types of programming for parishioners, such as classes on end-of-life issues, grief support groups, and help with special needs of hospitalized parishioners. The chaplain develops a relationship, as an institutional representative, with the parish nurse similar to those with other clergy in the community.

The chaplaincy department is a likely place for a nurse to seek personal learning opportunities that contribute to self-awareness and self-understanding. Often these needs go unmet since nurses are socialized to be other directed without a voice of their own (Stern and Spring, 1999). Clinical Pastoral Education (CPE) for nurses is an option (Nelson, 1995). Chaplaincy departments may offer special programs for volunteer lay chaplains and nurses can benefit from these programs also.

As coordinator of a large volunteer parish nurse program, this writer engaged a chaplain to teach "Equipping Lay Ministers," a program developed by a noted CPE supervisor, Dr. Ron Sunderland. Its purpose was to improve listening skills. Over a two-year period fifty-seven health ministers/parish nurses from a mission/ministry model completed the six-week program and thirty-two of them went on to complete a ten-week detailed experiential and didactic program on grief, loss, and transition issues. Program evaluations consistently reported that participants believed that they began to confront their own emotional baggage and to gain insight into themselves. They believe this is necessary before effectively responding to the spiritual needs of others.

Self-reflective educational process is typically not part of the nursing educational experience (Bevis, 1990; Yong, 1996). Student nurses usually are concerned with delivering the right intervention to the right patient at the right time; they neglect their own feelings and experiences during patient interactions. Nursing education does not encourage students to affirm their humanity as part of vocation formation and lacks an approach that reframes disappointments, stress, and discouragement into more positive perspectives (Wright, 1998).

In the mission/ministry model the parish nurse is the leader of the health ministry program of the parish and may go outside the parish to seek resources that will contribute to an effective ministry. The chaplain can provide specific services and follow alongside the ongoing ministry plan of the parish but would not be viewed as one to come in and "sell a new ministry" since the ministry goals arise from within the parish.

MARKETPLACE MODELS

The Parish Nurse

Positions are paid, usually through a health care organization. The nurse may or may not be a member of the parish. The church building becomes the site for delivery of health programs. Often the nurse, with knowledge of community health nursing concepts, is employed by health care partnerships and is a technical expert in the mobilization of resources for parishes. The nurse gathers data about what consumers want or need, implements programs, and interacts with bureaucracies.

Nurses may live out their faith while practicing in a marketplace program, but the underlying mission of the program reflects the employing organization. The employing health care institutions offer a product to a faith community, hopefully a culturally and faith-sensitive one. For instance, if a maternity clinic were provided in a Mexican community it would be good business to employ a nurse who could speak Spanish. Similarly, if a health product is being provided in a faith community, it is equally good business to employ a nurse who is familiar with that denomination or congregation.

Authority for the Parish Nurse Program

Marketplace models are usually connected in some way to health systems, operating through community outreach, chaplaincy, or other departments within a health system or nursing home. They are driven by economic values and offer a commodity to a consumer. Sometimes such parish nursing programs are a marketing or public relations tool. One such program exists as a collaborative partnership project between two competing hospitals as a demonstration of how they can work together effectively when resources are limited, contributing to a positive community image (White, 2000). Some institutions find parish nurse programs desirable simply because a competitive organization has such a program (Schumann, 2000). The efforts in some way contribute to the financial bottom line of a health system. Authority is determined in a negotiated arrangement between a parish and a health system. Marketplace models can offer in-reach programs for church members or outreach to underserved geographic neighbors of the sponsoring congregation.

Accountability in marketplace models is to the health system or funding agency. Some health systems offer services to parishes at no cost but expect photo options or publicity for their efforts; others negotiate a fee for services with the parish. Parishes can become involved in marketplace models in an effort to find a way to pay their parish nurse (Schuler, 2000) and these programs often impose strict standards for quantitative outcomes (Schumann, 2000). While persons may be served well by marketplace programs, the programs may in the end not be congruent with the ministry goals if parish leadership believes that ministry should originate from within the parish. Some faith traditions likely find it inappropriate to impose external regulations on their ministry.

Substance of the Parish Nurse Program

In marketplace programs, the community is viewed as a system of consumers with social or health problems that need to be solved by experts. The substance may be tied to a community indicator, such as high incidence of heart disease, or a calendar schedule, such as a different emphasis each month, e.g., heart month or diabetes month. The consumers can be individuals in parishes who want health programs on-site, parish groups that want to financially support a nurse to provide for the underserved, or partnerships that want to improve access to health care.

Health care is big business in the United States and health systems compete for their market share and goodwill in their communities. This competition can extend to the parish nurse program and questions emerge when reality does not reflect advertised claims. Church-based health services provided as a commodity do not necessarily translate into a ministry (Smith, 2000a). Some hospitals may use a parish nurse program to market their image in the community and parish clergy and health care chaplains need to recognize such endeavors for what they are.

Interface with Health Care Chaplains

In the 1990s, health systems discovered a market for spiritual care products because popular literature and scientific studies convinced many that religious practices improved health outcomes. Hospitals began to restore chaplaincy programs and sometimes placed parish nursing within them. Chaplains and nurses were challenged to work together.

From an academic perspective, the nurse is educated and socialized into a different meaning of spirituality than the chaplain (Wright,

1998). Spiritual development for the nurse is usually dependent on the commitment to one's faith traditions rather than the academic process. Chaplains in their seminary education and CPE reflect deeply on the meaning and purpose of life. Nursing education does not prepare nurses to undertake such in-depth reflection, to experience their feelings, and to learn things about themselves they would prefer not to recognize (Rolland, 1998). Parish nurses can benefit from chaplaincy programs that assist them in theological reflection on their own life stories in a contextual, unfolding process. Through narrative teaching methods chaplains can strengthen nurses in ministry formation (Nelson, 1995).

ACCESS MODELS

The Parish Nurse

The parish nurse is an advanced practice nurse specializing in community and public health nursing. As an advocate for the oppressed, the nurse is a catalyst or change agent to promote empowerment outcomes. Since the promotion of specific social justice issues can be problematic for some faith communities, the nurse who wishes to promote social change must carefully evaluate the ministry plan of a parish.

Authority for the Parish Nurse Program

Access models are often driven by philosophies of public health that offer services to societal victims, focusing on community development theories concerning advocacy, poverty, justice, and empowerment. The programs are often political in nature based on a philosophy that tries to realign existing resources between a dominant culture and the oppressed (Bracht, 1990; Freire, 1970; Perkins, 1995).

Access models emerged in response to the decline in accessible health care services and as governmental organizations began to seek community partners to assist with responsibilities of meeting the health care needs of the poor (Citrin, 1998). Positions are paid or unpaid. Many endowments and funding agencies will give grant monies to begin parish nursing programs that improve access to health care for the underserved as part of community coalitions. Faith can be expressed through access models because they will instill hope and teach that having a future is found in delaying instant gratification.

Substance of the Parish Nurse Program

These programs are developed from a generosity of spirit and a commitment to social justice. Generosity of spirit is an ability to acknowledge an interconnectedness—one's debts to society—that binds one to others (Bellah et al., 1985). The call is action based for a common good that leads to changes in the relationship between government and the economy. Program goals in this model seek to influence the political process and contribute to the recovery of social ecology. Individual goals focus on breaking downward spirals and hopelessness by helping the oppressed populations become self-sufficient and engaged in some way with a sense of direction for their own lives. Problem-solving education methods are valued since they affirm persons as beings in the process of becoming (Freire, 1970).

Interface with Health Care Chaplains

Interdisciplinary approaches require attention to integration rather than specialization, moving away from a divergent specialty toward a convergent integrated approach. As the nursing discipline has specialized over the years, nurses shifted from being generalists to becoming age specific, disease specific, site specific, gender specific, and role specific. Chaplains diverge in a similar fashion. Convergent approaches require coming together with less specialization and certain basic concepts from which to operate (McDaniel and Campbell, 1997; Panel Discussion, 1997; Smoot, Yancey, and Wagner, 1999). An integrated approach for parish nurses, chaplains, and parish clergy in the access model requires a public commitment to advocacy for social justice.

CONCLUSION

This chapter has described three models of parish nursing that may overlap in concrete situations. They constitute a theoretical lens through which the parish nurse, chaplain, and community clergy can clarify their aims and purposes as they come together for a health ministry.

In the mission/ministry model the client population includes the individuals and families served by the faith community and the power structure is the parish. The marketplace model provides a commodity to a consumer with the power structure being the agency to which the nurse or chaplain reports outcomes. In the access model, services are provided to victims of society and the power structure is political.

Parish nursing as a subspecialty of a secular discipline continues to emerge as a grassroots movement. Many programs exist as blends of these models and all three models make a contribution in their own way. The three professions must carefully evaluate which model(s) serves them best.

REFERENCES

Auerswald, E.H. (1968). Interdisciplinary versus ecological approach. *Family Process, 7*(2), 202-215.

Bakken, K.L. (1987). *The call to wholeness: Health as a spiritual journey.* New York: Crossroads.

Beckmen, R.J. (1995). *Praying for healing and wholeness.* Minneapolis: Augsburg Fortress.

Bellah, R.N., Madsen, R., Sullivan, W.M., Swidler, A., and Tipton, S.M. (1985). *Habits of the Heart.* New York: Harper and Row.

Bevis, E.O. (1990). Teaching and learning. In E.O. Bevis and J. Watson (Eds.), *Toward a caring curriculum: A new pedagogy for nursing* (pp. 153-187). National League for Nursing Publications. No. 15-2278.

Bracht, N. (1990). *Health promotion at the community level.* Newbury Park, CA: Sage Publications.

Buckhart, L. (1997). How to code nursing practice using NANDA and NIC. *Proceedings of the eleventh annual Westberg Parish Nurse Symposium,* Itasca, IL, 113-126.

Citrin, T. (1998). Topics of our times: Community or commodity. *American Journal of Public Health, 88*(3), 351-352.

Davis, L.L. (1997). What comes around doesn't necessarily go around. *Families, Systems, and Health, 15*(4), 401-404.

Friere, P. (1970). *Pedagogy of the oppressed.* New York: Herder and Herder.

Health Ministries Association and American Nurses Association (1998). *Scope and standards of parish nursing practice.* Washington, DC: American Nurses Publishing.

Magilvy, J.K. and Brown, N.J. (1997). Parish nursing: Advanced practice nursing: Model for healthier communities. *Advanced Practice Nursing Quarterly, 2*(4), 67-72.

McClosky, J.C. (1997). Nursing interventions classification: Defining nursing care. *Proceedings of the eleventh annual Westberg Parish Nurse Symposium*, Itasca, IL, 11-17.

McDaniel, S.H. and Campbell, T.L. (1997). Training health professionals to collaborate. *Families, Systems, and Health, 15*(4), 353-360.

Miller, L.W. (1997). Nursing through the lens of faith: A conceptual model. *Journal of Christian Nursing, 14*(1), 17-21.

Nelson, B. (1995). *Igniting the flame*. Bristol, ID: Wyndham Hall Press.

Panel Discussion (1997). Building community: Developing skills for interprofessional health professions education and relationship-centered care. *Families, Systems, and Health, 15*(4), 393-400.

Perkins, J.M. (1995). *Restoring at-risk communities: Doing it together and doing it right*. Grand Rapid, MI: Baker House.

Rolland, R.S. (1998). Beliefs and collaboration in illness: Evolution over time. *Families, Systems, and Health, 16*(½), 7-25.

Rydholm, L. (1997). Outcome based charting. *Proceedings of the eleventh annual Westberg Parish Nurse Symposium*, Itasca, IL, 19-26.

Schein, E.H. (1972). *Professional education*. New York: McGraw-Hill.

Schuler, L. (2000). Parish nursing is ministry. *Journal of Christian Nursing, 17*(1), 23.

Schumann, R. (2000). Collaboration for mission. *Journal of Christian Nursing, 17*(1), 22-23.

Smith, S.D. (1999). Response: Nursing in churches. *Insights, Austin Seminary Faculty Journal, 114*(2), 29-32.

Smith, S.D. (2000a). Parish nursing: A call to integrity. *Journal of Christian Nursing, 17*(1), 18-20.

Smith, S. D. (2000b). Practice models and educational pathways for parish nursing. *Oates Journal, 3* (Online: <http://www.oates.org/journal/mbr/vol-03-2000/articles/s_Smith-01.htm>).

Smoot, F.L., Yancey, V.J., and Wagner, T.J. (1999). An interdisciplinary approach to integrative professional education. *Journal of Pastoral Care, 53*(2), 153-160.

Stern, M.B. and Spring, N.M. (1999). Nurse abuse? Couldn't be! *Nurse Advocate* (Online: <www.nurseadvocate.org>).

Westberg, G. (1990). A historical perspective: Wholistic health and the parish nurse. In A. Solari-Twadell, A.M. Djupe, and M.A. McDermott (Eds.), *Parish nursing: The developing practice*. Park Ridge, IL: The National Parish Nurse Resource Center.

White, B.J. (2000). Pragmatic partnership. *Journal of Christian Nursing, 17*(1), 21-22.

Wright, K.B. (1998). Professional, ethical, and legal implications for spiritual care in nursing. *Image, 30*(1), 81-83.

Yong, V. (1996). "Doing clinical": The lived experience of nursing students. *Contemporary Nurse, 5*(2), 73-79.

SECTION VII:
FURTHER COOPERATION
AND RESOURCES FOR GROWTH

Chapter 19

Good Care of Patients: A Plea for More Humility and Less Pride from All Professionals

Pat Fosarelli

It may seem unusual for a physician to embrace a team approach. My own profession of medicine is accused, rightly in some circumstances, of claiming total control of patient care. Because physicians have expertise in the treatment of many physical problems, this control seems, on the surface, to make sense. However, a more in-depth perspective that I briefly outline in the following raises serious questions about that view.

I am enthusiastic about the team approach because it acknowledges that individual perspectives are so limited that they require the assistance of others. The enormous complexity of another human being demands a response of humble acknowledgment of our limitations.

The team approach is necessary because the physical condition of patients always affects their emotional states. I argue that the converse holds true as well; emotional states affect physical conditions. Indeed, we now know that certain psychological states are likely to contribute to measurable positive or negative physiological changes. Furthermore, as more people are willing to discuss the spiritual aspect of their lives, it seems that the physical and the spiritual (not to mention the psychological and the spiritual) may be linked as well. Certainly we know that selected psychological states are related to certain spiritual states. For example, promising research results demonstrate that the act of praying or meditating is associated with the release of endorphins, those chemicals made by our own bodies which counteract the stress-evoked "fight-or-flight" response associated with increased blood pressure and diminished immune responses. Endorphin release, on the other hand, is associated with factors important to health such as lower blood pressure, lower heart rate, lower breathing rate, and improved immune responses.

Despite this knowledge, medical education and practice change very slowly. I remember one medical school professor telling us as medical students that asking about patient beliefs was like asking how they voted in the last election; it was completely irrelevant to patient care. Medical students learn virtually nothing about the spiritual dimension of patients even today. Of course, this dimension is invariably present, even if patients claim no particular religious affiliation or cannot acknowledge a personal spirituality.

We now know that the logic, to use the term quite loosely, of the medical school professor is tragically flawed. Beliefs may make a substantial difference between being overwhelmed with one's own problems and reaching out to others, between being plagued with chronic disabilities and learning to live with or in spite of them. Belief can influence the decision whether to get well or to die.

Other professionals are secondary if physicians are the absolute rulers of patient care. This dominance is expressed in actions, words, and attitudes. For example, no matter who is speaking with a patient, that person frequently defers to a physician who enters the room. A chaplain might say, "Oh, your doctor is here; I can come back" even when the discussion pertains to difficulties with adhering to medical regimens or to a perception that illness is God's will and to "escape" it is sinful. Such discussions have enormous implications for both doctors and patients and they ought to be continued when physicians enter the room. Similarly, community clergy usually move out of the way when a medical team enters the room, even though the medical students know far less about ill people than experienced pastors. What is needed is teamwork, not turf work.

I think that meaningful teamwork is possible among parish nurses, community clergy, and health care chaplains, but the usual turf issues also complicate these relationships. Who has the most knowledge and who is in charge? The pastor may know the patient's spiritual life best but may not understand the physical, emotional, and spiritual issues of the patient's current illness as well as the parish nurse. The health care chaplain may not have even met the patient previously. Last night, however, the patient learned the bad news from the surgery and the chaplain was called. They had a long heart-to-heart talk and the chaplain now has current insights about the patient's spiritual issues. In addition, health care chaplains know the institutional environment better than the parish nurse or pastor.

Other turf issues certainly emerge. Is team leadership a static arrangement or will it vary by patient or situation? Will it even vary for the same patient at different times in his or her illness? What happens when team members have widely divergent views on such theological issues as the power of prayer in healing, the importance of healing services, theodicy issues, or the nature of sin and punishment? One woman told me that she had asked to see a Catholic priest as she entered a hospital for surgery. A priest did not visit, but several days after her procedure, a priest whom she had never met entered her room and opened the conversation with, "When was your last confession?" before introducing himself or learning more about her. When she was at a loss for words, he said, "Well you know that illness is frequently punishment for sin." To whom does such a woman turn if she does not believe the priest's statement? After all, she is captive in a bed! The person visiting her was the hospital's Catholic chaplain who made the visit because her own pastor was away and the congregation had no parish nurse. In distress, the woman later called the nurse caring for her that day and sobbed. The nurse listened.

Spiritual crises arise frequently in the course of a hospitalization or during a protracted course of therapy for a chronic condition. Examples include persons struggling with the prospect of a surgical procedure or a bad diagnosis. Thus, some health professionals must be able to deal with spiritual concerns as part of their tasks. A parish nurse, by virtue of training in both nursing and theology, has an advantage that most health professionals and most clergy do not have.

This does not mean, however, that parish nurses always are in the best position to deal with spiritual struggles. First, the nurse's grasp of the person's current hospital situation may not be as good as that of the chaplain who spent the last evening with that patient and the family. Second, the patient may wish to talk with the pastor, a person with whom the patient may have a long-term relationship.

A patient's relationship to a pastor is frequently very important because the two share a history. Assuming the history is a positive one, the pastor may make valuable contributions to the patient's total care. If that history is negative or virtually nonexistent, the pastor may be a hindrance to the care. For example, the mother of one of my patients told me that she did not want the pastor to visit her child in the hospital. "He has judged me ever since I became HIV positive," she said. "He told me it was my wicked lifestyle. Fine. Now that my child is sick, I don't want to see his face and hear his voice in my baby's room." For other patients, the pastor may be almost a nonentity. "I never talked with our pastor," a father told me. "I mean, he was there at services, but he doesn't really know me or my family. Not enough to help, anyway." The father seemed unaware that this might be the occasion to build a relationship with the pastor.

Health care chaplains are frequently in a very awkward position because they do not meet the individual patient until the hospitalization or the crisis. They are meeting patients at perhaps the worst possible time, certainly not a time when they are at their best. Yet, patients frequently welcome chaplains because they will not examine them, draw blood, or perform another procedure. But not everyone welcomes chaplains. Some assume that the visit means "God talk" when they are most vulnerable. They refuse the visit because they do not believe in God, are angry at God or the Church (because of the action of a minister or church member, perhaps even years before), or fear that the present illness is God's judgment of their lives up to this point. Some patients take exception to certain chaplains because of their gender or race. A chaplain might remind a patient of the clergy who reprimanded the patient in eighth grade or who questioned the patient during a period of excesses in younger years. Such concerns easily rise to the surface when patients are stressed and vulnerable.

Tragically, turf battles are sometimes fought over the beds of patients. Patients have commented to me that their clergy criticized a chaplain or vice versa. More recently, as parish nursing has emerged, patients have noted that parish nurses sometimes take issue with the pastor or the chaplain. Each professional may truly believe that he or she has the best interests of patients at heart. Each may truly believe that he or she is professionally correct in his or her approach, but these difficulties should not be debated in front of patients.

Thus, each team member brings potential strengths and liabilities to every patient encounter. Strengths can be maximized only by laying aside turf issues and working as a team for the good of a given patient. A parish nurse cannot always say, "I'm both health professional and minister. Because I understand both areas, follow my lead." The pastor cannot always say, "I'm the pastor, and because I know this person's spiritual life better than everyone else, follow my lead." The chaplain cannot always say, "I've seen these situations a hundred times in my career. Because I know what people are going through in such circumstances, follow my lead." Although each of the premises may well be true for each of the professionals, the conclusions do not necessarily follow.

The best time for meaningful dialogue is before a crisis. These professionals in the team must reach agreement before the crisis on how they will provide ministry to their ill or hospitalized congregants. This is not to suggest a cookbook approach because each congregant is different, but their ongoing knowledge of the patient and family can inform their decisions.

Community clergy, parish nurses, and health care chaplains will function better together if they respect one another. Monthly or quarterly meetings, breakfasts, or luncheons can be opportunities to talk. Many professionals use such meetings for educational enrichment, but they must also talk with one another to know where they agree and where they disagree. That is precisely why lectures alone do not promote fellowship; attendees are so busy taking notes or asking questions that they do not have the time to get to know one another and learn why others think differently than they do.

Time is of the essence. These professionals live very complex lives. The demands on their time and energy are enormous. They face suffering each day, and they must learn to work with that suffering for the benefit of those to whom they minister. Retreats (or "quiet time") designed for all three groups, even if only for a morning or an afternoon, permit all present to appreciate one another's vulnerability and limitations. They also have the opportunity to witness one another's gifts and marvel how God provides. Getting to know one another tears down any chance of an "us versus them" mentality, as all struggle to live as God wants them to live for the good of others.

Can doctors also be part of such teamwork? Is it possible for parish nurses, chaplains, and pastors to have a healthy attitude about doctors and vice versa? I believe so, but only if all concerned are willing to dialogue and share experiences—not as experts but as fellow ministers to the people of God. Many doctors must learn to regard parish nurses, community clergy, and chaplains as essential rather than superfluous to the care of a patient. They must appreciate that spiritual concerns will impact the physical and psychological states of many patients; they must have the proper respect for that spiritual aspect of the human person, even if they themselves do not understand it. Conversely, parish nurses, chaplains, and community clergy must learn to view doctors as skilled professionals who have gifts and limitations. They must avoid the temptation either to denigrate physicians or to lionize them because both views are unfair. Each must see the other as a member of the same team. This is important not only from a practical point of view ("get the patient better") but also from spiritual and moral viewpoints which remind all members of the team that they have limitations and that the patient and God are also members of that team. Indeed, the God whose children we all are has given each of us particular gifts for our respective ministries. Instead of vying with one another, we are called to celebrate these gifts and welcome their inclusion into the total care of those to whom we are privileged to minister.

Chapter 20

Resources for Individual
and Team Growth

Richard B. Gilbert

The broom of change has swept across American culture, leaving no corner, no pathway, no sacred foundation untouched. Everything is questioned, scrutinized, as we ask whether it offers any meaning or truth for this new millennium. Religion, generally, and the church, specifically, are not spared. In contrast, spiritual hunger is rampant and authors demonstrate an outburst of interest by producing materials that introduce spiritual language and values to institutions, workplaces, and social intercourse. Web sites blossom, spiritual rituals emerge, and people continue to profess, in high numbers, a belief in God.

As we witness an increased commitment to spirituality and spiritual matters, growing suspicion of religion and a decline in religious or corporate participation continues. While it varies from denomination to denomination and parish to parish, a bit more than 50 percent of Americans now indicate that religion is no longer relevant or helpful.

Social theologians speak of spirituality and culture. In terms of the church we speak of a paradigm shift, moving from the church of today to the church of tomorrow. This has generated enthusiasm and creative energy for some; many others experience fear or resistance and a return to dynamics of control, power, codependency, and dysfunction.

In the midst of this storm of change we see clergy asking, "Who am I?" "What is my call to ministry?" and "What is being asked of me?" The conflicts of society have become the conflicts of the church. New interest in spirituality and spiritual care in health care has redefined (and, in some centers, crushed) pastoral care. Growth in lay ministries, often with national training centers, has diminished ordained ministry in its present form. Many clergy are leaving; others have developed personal, emotional, or family problems. Many flounder, asking these essential questions of identity and purpose.

While many suggest that the religious voice has been silenced in America, or at least is taken less seriously, more and more people are turning to religious institutions for care and support. Managed care, especially in areas of mental health, has increased burdens for individuals who now must find alternative sources for care. Clergy are being asked to become "experts" in more and more social issues and human predicaments, often with little or no training and frequently at their own peril. Legislators look for ways to slash budgets and attack funding for the frequently marginalized. They even suggest that "the churches will fill the gap."

What is parish ministry today? In many ways it consists of redefined roles; unclear visions; increased expectations placed on time, struggles to balance self, job, and family; and the need for more programming and staff without increased budgets. Often parishioners do not understand these changes.

It is also an exciting time to create, dream, take risks, and be innovative. What did not work yesterday may well work today. One of the most exciting and visionary developments is in the role of the parish nurse. It brings an ally for ministers, a skilled clinician to be an extension of parish leadership, and a professional committed to holistic values and rights that bring gospel to people and people to gospel in ways previously unknown. It is amazing how spiritual matters can come forth while a blood pressure is checked, a home visit is made, or an assessment is completed.

This development has not come easily. Many parish nurses either volunteer or are underpaid. Some clergy are threatened by anyone and anything that appears to put pressure on their kingdoms. We are aware of these dynamics, but we must not let them stop us. Programs and teams will grow through our commitment to parish nursing, along with the hard work of training, study, personal care, and spiritual discernment.

Continuing education is mandatory. This will not be welcome news for some clergy. Many clergy limit themselves to occasional workshops on often repetitive subjects presented by denominational leaders even further removed from the realities of ministry. Seminaries cannot bear the entire load for clergy development, at least with current funding levels. Clergy need to develop skills in the following: personal spirituality, bereavement care, crisis intervention, domestic violence awareness, and much more. Such skills continue to speak in relevant and meaningful ways to today's issues. Continuing education cannot be limited to workshops on stewardship, evangelism, and preaching the lectionary. Clergy must integrate continuing education, thoughtfully prepared with accountability to parish and denominational leadership, into their ongoing professional growth. Congregations or denominations must also stress the importance of continuing education and provide the funds to address these needs.

Nurses have long known the importance of continuing education and professional development around their professional and licensing needs. They now are integrating new dimensions of nursing previously untouched due to the rush of managed care, including a growing respect for spirituality (which has always been a priority for nursing). This keeps before them the challenge to see the holistic approach to care and also to remember that the heart of ministry, in any form, is about presence. Presence does not fit neatly and tidily into the medical model; presence is about listening to people and their stories.

This brings us to the contents of this chapter—reading resources that will encourage new thinking. The resources are organized in three sections. Crossover (in the first two) is encouraged so that clergy can learn about parish nursing, and vice versa. The third section is a very introductory resource list to the broader sweep of pastoral care and the needs of people. Our World Pastoral Care Center remains available to you for training, support, certification, and help with resources. We can be contacted at 847-429-2110, dick.gilbert@shermanhospital.org or at <www.twpcc.org>. For other resource assistance on parish nursing you are also invited to contact the resource center at the International Parish Nurse Center, The Deaconess Center, 475 E. Lockwood, St. Louis, MO 63119, 314-918-2527 or <http://ipnrc.parishnurses.org>.

FOR AND ABOUT PASTORS AND PASTORAL CARE

Brother John of Taize. *The Adventure of Holiness: Biblical Foundations and Present-Day Perspectives.* New York: Alba House, 1999.
  Rediscovering the call and authority for ministry.

Butler, Sarah A. *Caring Ministry: A Contemplative Approach to Pastoral Care.* New York: Continuum, 1999.

>   *An outstanding read, a confident blending of pastoral care with centered living and prayer. A good compendium of resources to train lay ministers and seminarians.*

Carr, Wesley. *Handbook of Pastoral Studies.* London: SPCK, 1997.

>   *One of the most insightful, persuasive and encouraging studies available on pastoral care and pastoral caregivers.*

Cetuk, Virginia Samuel. *What to Expect in Seminary: Theological Education as Spiritual Formation.* Nashville, TN: Abingdon Press, 1998.

>   *Grinds us to a halt in the assembly line of ministry formation by asking what formation can and should be.*

Coate, Mary Anne. *Clergy Stress: The Hidden Conflicts in Ministry.* London: SPCK, 1989.

>   *A very wise friend in leading us through the stresses and strains of ministry.*

Copenhaver, Martin B., Anthony B. Robinson, and William H. Willimon. *Good News in Exile: Three Pastors Offer a Hopeful Vision for the Church.* Grand Rapids, MI: Eerdmans, 1999.

>   *A timely rebirthing for congregations, denominations, and those who minister in and to them.*

Countryman, L. William. *Living On the Border of the Holy: Renewing the Priesthood of All.* Harrisburg, PA: Morehouse Publishing, 1999.

>   *A book about and for clergy, people "who live in the dangerous, exhilarating, life-giving borderlands of human existence." Timely, applicable.*

Dorff, Francis. *The Journey from Misery to Ministry; Living Creatively in a Broken World.* Notre Dame, IN: Ave Maria Press, 1998.

>   *Moving us from the stagnant to the lively, from the miserable and unhealthy to the healthy and creative.*

Gilbert, Richard. *Responding to Grief: A Complete Resource Guide.* Point Richmond, CA: Spirit of Health!, 1997.

>   *Over 1,000 titles (books, cassettes, videos), sixty subjects, plus information on agencies, publishers, and programs.*

Greeley, Andrew. *Furthermore! Memories of a Parish Priest.* New York: Forge, 1999.

This skilled storyteller uses story, instruction, and honesty to bring us close to who and what is a parish minister.

Hover, Margot. *Caring for Yourself When Caring for Others.* Mystic, CT: Twenty-Third Publications, 1994.

A rare, healthy, and rigorous look at who we are, what we do, and how we must be responsible for taking care of ourselves.

Jacobs, Michael. *Still Small Voice: An Introduction to Pastoral Counselling.* London: SPCK, 1982.

A very practical look at pastoral care and counseling skills, refuting the impracticalities we often bring to the context.

Langford, Daniel L. *The Pastor's Family: The Challenges of Family Life and Pastoral Responsibilities.* Binghamton, NY: The Haworth Pastoral Press, 1998.

Meyer, Chuck. *Dying Church Living God: A Call to Begin Again.* Kelowna, British Columbia, Canada: Northstone, 2000.

Blending mystery, contemporary imagery, scripture, and personal experience we have a prophetic and pastoral look at the church, the marginalized, and the ministers, themselves among the marginalized.

Niklas, Gerald. *The Making of a Pastoral Person* (Expanded and Revised Edition). New York: Alba House, 1996.

Hospital chaplains are in a special place to bring care and insight to those in the parish. This book offers these insights in a brilliant way.

Nouwen, Henri. *The Wounded Healer.* Garden City, NY: Image Books, 1972.

Where all study and discussion of ministry begins.

Oates, Wayne E. *Confessions of a Workaholic: The Facts About Work Addiction.* Nashville, TN: Abingdon Press, 1971.

We naively believe we can never do too much for God and ministry and find ourselves on the path to self-destruction. This book is essential.

O'Meara, Thomas F. *Theology of Ministry* (Revised Edition). Mahwah, NJ: Paulist Press, 1999.

> *While offering a unique view of ministry within the Roman Catholic Church, the book is rich in the theology of ministry for all denominations.*

Oswald, Roy M. *Clergy Self-Care; Finding a Balance for Effective Ministry.* Washington, DC: Alban Institute, 1991.

> *We talk about setting priorities and clarifying boundaries. It feels like walking a very thin tightrope while juggling too many expectations, goals, and demands. An important book.*

Owens, Virginia Stem. *Looking for Jesus.* Louisville, KY: Westminster John Knox Press, 1998.

> *By sharing the stories and personalities of the Bible we learn about ourselves, our faith, and our practice.*

Pattison, Stephen. *A Critique of Pastoral Care.* London: SCM, 1988.

> *Asks the question "What is pastoral care anyway?" and, in a structured and content-rich way, leads us to a meaningful reply.*

Perri, William D. *A Radical Challenge for Priesthood Today: From Trial to Transformation.* Mystic, CT: Twenty-Third Publications, 1996.

> *These are radical times that demand radical clergy with a radical gospel.*

Peterson, James. *More I Could Not Ask: Finding Christ in the Margins (a Priest's Story).* New York: Crossroad, 1999.

> *In the margins we meet Christ, the marginalized, ourselves in the margins, and the work we call ministry.*

Rediger, G. Lloyd. *Clergy Killers: Guidance for Pastors and Congregations Under Attack.* Louisville, KY: Westminster John Knox Press, 1997.

> *A tragic but honest look at what ministry frequently becomes.*

Ritter, Kathleen and Craig O'Neill. *Righteous Religion: Unmasking the Illusions of Fundamentalism and Authoritarian Catholicism.* Binghamton, NY: The Haworth Pastoral Press, 1996.

> *It is not about specific denominations or teachings, but common and dangerous practices that bring out the abusive worst in congregations, individuals, judicatories, and clergy. This book needs to be read.*

Roberts, Wes. *Support Your Local Pastor: Practical Ways to Encourage Your Minister.* Colorado Springs, CO: Navpress, 1995.

> *Designed for parishioners and parish leaders to help them welcome their new minister, it is a very helpful look at what parish ministry is about and how to keep it healthy. Some important reminders for clergy readers are included.*

Smith, Karen Sue. *Priesthood in the Modern World: A Reader.* Franklin, WI: Sheed and Ward, 1999.

> *A very diverse collection of essays that cut to the heart of what ministry is and what it can and must be. Very thoughtful and pastoral.*

Steere, David A. *Spiritual Presence in Psychotherapy: A Guide for Caregivers.* New York: Brunner/Mazel, 1997.

> *A very thorough look at the work of clergy as counselors and the relationship between counseling and spirituality. Enhances skills; helps us keep our boundaries clear.*

Sweetser, Thomas P., S.J. McKinney and Mary Benet McKinney. *Changing Pastors: A Resource for Pastoral Transitions.* Kansas City: Sheed and Ward, 1998.

> *Few things present more risk, challenge, and opportunity for congregations and leadership than the change of pastoral leadership. This book is a helpful, step-by-step friend to parish leaders, members, and pastors.*

Walmsley, Roberta Chapin and Adair T. Lummis. *Healthy Clergy Wounded Healers: Their Families and Their Ministries.* New York: Church Publishing, 1997.

> *A very careful and critical study of how we call, train, and support our clergy and also the impact of ministry on the family.*

Zikmund, Barbara Brown, Adair T. Lummis, and Patricia Mei Yin Chang. *Clergy Women: An Uphill Calling.* Louisville, KY: Westminster John Knox Press, 1998.

> *A novel look at women in ministry, men in ministry . . . and ministry.*

Zurheide, Jeffry. *When Faith Is Tested: Pastoral Responses to Suf-fering and Tragic Death.* Minneapolis, MN: Augsburg Fortress Press, 1997.

> *While it is intended to awaken clergy to the needs of the be-reaved, it also introduces us to our own bereaved needs and what pastoral care must be.*

FOR AND ABOUT PARISH NURSES

We have only listed books. You are encouraged to do an article search. In addition, the book that accompanies the annual parish nurse symposium is available from the International Parish Nurse Resource Center listed previously.

Djupe, Anne Marie. *Looking Back, the Parish Nurse Experience (Phase 1 Report): A Summary of the Structure, Resources, Goals, Activities and Accomplishments of 40 Parish Nurse Programs.* Park Ridge, IL: Parish Nurse Resource Center, 1992.

Djupe, Anne Marie. *Reaching Out—Parish Nursing Services: An In-stitutionally Based Model of Parish Nursing Services.* Park Ridge, IL: Parish Nurse Resource Center, 1994.

> *A helpful look at the many ways (and settings) that parish nurses can serve.*

Kinast, Robert and Larry Seidl. *Partners in Healing: Healthcare Or-ganizations and Parish Communities.* St. Louis, KY: Catholic Health, 1996.

> *A visionary work, bringing together congregations and institu-tions around common values and goals through shared visions and ministries.*

Nelson, Barbara. *Igniting the Flame: Clinical Pastoral Education for Nurses.* Bristol, PA: Wyndham Hall, 1992.

> *CPE has its stars and its scars, but it is a powerful approach to integrating self-holistically so that holistic care can follow. It brings nurses into a common ground with many in ministry.*

Sharpe, William. *Medicine and the Ministry: A Medical Basis for Pastoral Care.* New York: Appleton-Century, 1966.

> *Although the book predates much of contemporary health care delivery, it gives us solid definitions and frameworks for mea-suring effectiveness.*

Shelly, Judy and Arlene Miller. *Called to Care*. Downers Grove, IL: Intervarsity Press, 1999.

> *A very thorough development of a Christian paradigm for nursing and nurses.*

Shortell, S.M., R.R. Gillies, D.A. Anderson, K.M. Erickson, and J.B. Mitchell. *Remaking Healthcare in America: Building Organized Delivery Systems*. San Francisco, CA: Jossey-Bass, 1996.

> *An important broad-based look at contemporary health care delivery, providing a context for ministry and quality care.*

Solari-Twadell, Phyllis Ann and Mary Ann McDermott. *Parish Nursing: Promoting Whole Person Health Within Faith Communities*. Thousand Oaks, CA: Sage, 1999.

> *This will serve as the authoritative work on parish nursing for many years to come. A diverse collection of essays.*

Westberg, Granger and Jill Westberg McNamara. *Parish Nurse: Providing a Minister of Health for Your Congregation*. Minneapolis, MN: Augsburg Fortress: 1990.

> *Building on their earlier founding work, we have additional direction on team and program building.*

Westberg, Granger with Jill Westberg McNamara. *The Parish Nurse: How to Start a Parish Nurse Program in Your Church*. Park Ridge, IL: Parish Nurse Resource Center, 1987.

> *The birthing book, the spirit, and the mission of parish nursing.*

SPECIFIC OPPORTUNITIES FOR MINISTRY: FOR MINISTERS AND NURSES

Aging

Felber, Marta. *Grief Expressed When a Mate Dies*. West Fork, AK: Life Words, 1997.

> *A hands-on approach to helping the widowed deal with their losses and guide themselves through this time of transition. A good guide for professionals who seek to provide support.*

Grollman, Earl with Sharon Grollman. *Your Aging Parents: Reflections for Caregivers*. Boston: Beacon Press, 1999.

> *A very helpful guide for adults dealing with their aging parents. Strong awareness of spiritual concerns.*

Grollman, Earl with Kenneth Kosik. *When Someone You Love Has Alzheimer's: The Caregiver's Journey.* Boston: Beacon Press, 1996.

> *Written for those closest to those suffering with Alzheimer's, themselves suffering, this book is equally informative for professionals who must strive to eliminate the isolation that accompanies this journey.*

Jones, Doris Moreland. *And Not One Bird Stopped Singing: Coping with Transition and Loss in Aging.* Nashville, TN: Upper Room Books, 1997.

> *The aging find and claim hope, story, and self-worth.*

Kirkland, Kevin and Howard McIlveen. *Full Circle: Spiritual Therapy for the Elderly.* Binghamton, NY: The Haworth Press, Inc., 1999.

> *An important text for professionals that includes definitions, rationale, discussion of feelings, life review, and dealing with special occasions and spiritual concerns.*

Koenig, Harold G. *Aging and God: Spiritual Pathways to Mental Health in Midlife and Later Years.* Binghamton, NY: The Haworth Press, Inc., 1994.

> *A very important collection of readings on a variety of related subjects.*

Koenig, Harold G. and Andrew J. Weaver. *Pastoral Care of Older Adults.* Minneapolis: Augsburg Fortress, 1998.

> *Not to be limited to pastors, includes several essays on subjects such as aging and physical health, facilitating spiritual growth, locating community resources, when a nursing home becomes necessary, dealing with disability or dependency, etc.*

McCall, Junietta Baker. *Grief Education for Caregivers of the Elderly.* Binghamton, NY: The Haworth Press, Inc., 1999.

> *A good discussion of bereavement issues unique to the aging, and also program assistance for providing quality support.*

Morgan, John D. *Ethical Issues in the Care of the Dying and Bereaved Aged.* Amityville, NY: Baywood, 1996.

> *With this book you have one of the best collections of essays with a very diverse approach to the subject. Essential.*

Oates, Wayne E. *Grief, Transition, and Loss: A Pastor's Practical Guide.* Minneapolis, MN: Augsberg Fortress Press, 1997.

In addition to grief associated with death, this book also discusses loss and divorce, separation, and work-related losses.

Siegal, Alan and Robert Siegal. *Forget Me Not: Caring for and Coping with Your Aging Parents.* Berkeley, CA: Celestial Arts, 1993.

A helpful discussion of the struggles experienced by adult children called upon to deal with aging parents and with themselves.

Sullender, R. Scott. *Losses in Later Life: A New Way of Walking with God* (Second Edition). Binghamton, NY: The Haworth Press, Inc., 1999.

Linking aging, loss, and the resources of spirit and Spirit.

Sunderland, Ron. *Getting Through Grief Caregiving by Congregations.* Nashville, TN: Abingdon Press, 1993.

Sunderland is the best for mobilizing congregations for planned action to address a personal or community need. Includes discussion of losses in addition to those associated with a death.

VandeCreek, Larry. *Spiritual Care for Persons with Dementia: Fundamentals for Pastoral Practice.* Binghamton, NY: The Haworth Press, Inc., 1999.

Speaks forcefully about those suffering with dementia and to all of us who must walk with them, often without addressing our own issues, fears, and uncertainties.

Weaver, Andrew, Harold Koenig, and Phyllis Roe. *Reflections on Aging and Spiritual Growth.* Nashville, TN: Abingdon Press, 1998.

Stories, instruction, meditations, resources.

Bereavement

DeSpelder, Lynne Ann and Albert Lee Strickland. *The Last Dance: Encountering Death and Dying* (Fifth Edition). Mountain View, CA: Mayfield Publishing, 1999.

Considered by many to be the most authoritative textbook and reference guide on matters related to dying, death, and bereavement.

Gilbert, Richard. *HeartPeace: Healing Help for Grieving Folks.* St. Meinrad, IN: Abbey Press, 1996.

> *Brief, gentle, to the point. A rare look at the interdependence between bereavement and spirituality. Excellent as a gift item for the bereaved.*

Gilbert, Richard. *Responding to Grief: A Complete Resource Guide.* Point Richmond, CA: Spirit of Health!, 1997. (Two supplements available directly from the author.)

> *Packed. Over 1,000 titles of books, videos, cassettes, brochures, divided into sixty subjects, with instruction and other resource information.*

Gilbert, Richard. *Finding Your Way When Your Parent Dies: Hope for Adult Children.* Notre Dame, IN: Ave Maria Press, 1999.

> *A significant look, with spiritual care, at a loss that comes to all of us, and the significance of which is often diminished. Can also be used for counseling and class discussion.*

Grollman, Earl A. *Straight Talk About Death For Teenagers.* Boston: Beacon Press, 1993.

> *The best book for teenagers and for those who work with them.*

Grollman, Earl A. *Bereaved Children and Teens: A Support Guide for Parents and Professionals.* Boston: Beacon Press, 1995.

> *A very good collection of essays for those who work with children, including several that discuss spiritual matters and faith traditions.*

Grollman, Earl A. *Living When a Loved One Has Died.* Boston: Beacon Press, 1995.

> *The one book to have and to give away.*

Gryte, Marilyn. *No New Baby: For Siblings Who Have a Brother or Sister Die Before Birth.* Omaha, NB: Centering, 1998.

> *Sibling loss—easily misunderstood or forgotten. A fine gift book for young children confronted by the loss of a sibling during pregnancy.*

Hope for Bereaved. *Hope for Bereaved.* Syracuse, NY: Hope for Bereaved, Inc., 1995.

A collection of some sixty first-person articles that teach and comfort—on a wide variety of subjects. A must-have book for your library.

Hutchison, Joyce and Joyce Rupp. *May I Walk You Home? Courage and Comfort for Caregivers of the Very Ill.* Notre Dame, IN: Ave Maria Press, 1999.

A rare find. For the loved ones of the seriously ill and also for the professionals who surround them.

Meyer, Charles. *A Good Death: Challenges, Choices and Care Options.* Mystic, CT: Twenty-Third Publications, 1999.

Speaks of the possibility of a "good death," and the practicalities (and hope) for the dying, their loved ones and those professionally involved.

Moe, Thomas. *Pastoral Care in Pregnancy Loss: A Ministry Long Needed.* Binghamton, NY: The Haworth Press, Inc., 1997.

A loss steeped in spiritual concerns and pastoral needs, yet often faced alone.

Morgan, John D. *Readings in Thanatology.* Amityville, NY: Baywood, 1997.

Over twenty-five essays contributed by some of the best in the field, including North American death attitudes, caring for the terminally ill, bereavement, children and death, questions of values, and suicide.

O'Brien, Mauryeen. *Praying Through Grief: Healing Prayer Services for Those Who Mourn.* Notre Dame, IN: Ave Maria Press, 1997.

A gentle weaving through loss by means of rituals that serve for individual family use, for families, and for congregational life and health.

Oliver, Samuel. *What the Dying Teach Us.* Binghamton, NY: The Haworth Press, Inc., 1998.

What the dying can teach us (if we will listen) and what we have to offer them.

Wezeman, Phyllis Vos, Jude Dennis Fournier, and Kenneth R. Wezeman. *Guiding Children Through Life's Losses: Prayers, Rituals and Activities.* Mystic, CT: Twenty-Third Publications, 1998.

> *Excellent resource guide and befriender at times of need and also for the ongoing life and needs of congregations, families, and children.*

The Sick

DeGildio, Sandra. *Praying with the Sick: Prayers, Services, Rituals.* Mystic, CT: Twenty-Third Publications, 1998.

> *Buy it in quantity, for your use, for lay ministers, for families/loved ones, and for the sick.*

Dexter, Pat Egan. *Coping As Caregivers: When a Loved One Is Ill.* Mystic, CT: Twenty-Third Publications, 1999.

> *A friendly help to friends providing love, care, and support.*

Glen, Genevieve, Marilyn Kofler, and Kevin O'Connor. *Handbook for Ministers of Care* (Second Edition). Chicago: Liturgical Training Publications, 1997.

> *A good training resource for various types of lay ministries in various settings.*

Grollman, Earl. *Caring and Coping When Your Loved One Is Seriously Ill.* Boston: Beacon Press, 1995.

> *This is a book you can place in the hands of struggling loved ones.*

Guntzelman, Joan. *125 Prayers for Caregivers.* Winona, MN: Saint Mary's Press, 1995.

> *One hundred twenty-five reasons to have—and use—this book.*

Miller, James. *The Caregiver's Book: Caring for Another, Caring for Yourself.* Fort Wayne, IN: Willowgreen, 1996.

> *Miller has a rare gift, blending words, pictures, and comfort.*

Vanderzee, John. *Ministry to Persons with Chronic Illnesses: A Guide to Empowerment Through Negotiation.* Minneapolis, MN: Augsburg Fortress Press, 1993.

> *The authority on chronic illness.*

Counseling, Emotional Support, Mental Health

Jacobs, Michael. *Still Small Voice: An Introduction to Pastoral Counseling.* London: SPCK, 1982.

One of many good introductions to pastoral care, with definitions, discussion of key issues, and resource information.

Koenig, Harold G. *Is Religion Good for Your Health? The Effects of Religion on Physical and Mental Health.* Binghamton, NY: The Haworth Press, Inc., 1997.

Give it a careful read. Important information that will guide you in your work.

McBride, J. LeBron. *Spiritual Crisis: Surviving Trauma to the Soul.* Binghamton, NY: The Haworth Press, Inc., 1998.

Brings us directly into the experience we call crisis and its impact on belief and the ability to believe.

Oates, Wayne. *Behind the Masks: Personality Disorders in Religious Behavior.* Louisville, KY: Westminster John Knox Press, 1987.

Gives definitions, assessment tools and skills for dealing with emotional crises that either result from religious issues or directly affect them.

Parad, Howard and Libbie Parad, editors. *Crisis Intervention Book 2: The Practitioner's Sourcebook for Brief Therapy.* Milwaukee, WI: Family Service America, 1990.

A compendium of theory, technologies, and clinical practices around many life experiences. Written by experts in the field. Brief essays to the point.

Whitehead, James D. and Evelyn Eaton Whitehead. *Shadows of the Heart: A Spirituality of the Negative Emotions.* New York: Crossroad, 1994.

Useful reference guide around "negative" emotions and their impact on people. Assessment tools and clinical practice.

Whitehead, James D. and Evelyn Eaton Whitehead. *Shadows of the Heart: A Spirituality of the Painful Emotions.* New York: Crossroad, 1994.

Includes discussion of befriending our emotions, emergency emotions, shame and guilt, and transforming our emotions.

Domestic Violence

Fall, Kevin, Shareen Howard, and June Ford. *Alternatives to Domestic Violence: A Homework Manual for Battering Intervention Groups.* Philadelphia, PA: Accelerated Development, 1999.

> *Experts in the field consider this an outstanding book—especially useful in helping churches confront a significant denial: there is domestic violence in every congregation.*

Schornstein, Sherri L. *Domestic Violence and Health Care: What Every Professional Needs to Know.* Thousand Oaks, CA: Sage, 1997.

> *Good demographics, statistics, definitions, plus a thorough integration of institutional concerns that enable us to build bridges to the community and to parishes. Amply points out areas where the medical system contributes to the problem rather than serves as part of the solution.*

Addiction

Apthorp, Stephen. *Alcohol and Substance Abuse: A Clergy Handbook.* Harrisburg, PA: Morehouse, 1985.

> *Not only is it very thorough in what it teaches about addiction, but also addresses clergy/pastoral care blindness to the presence of addiction in the congregation and our drivenness commonly rooted in codependent behaviors on our part.*

Booth, Leo. *Spirituality and Recovery: A Guide to Positive Living.* Deerfield Beach, FL: Health Communications, 1988.

> *Extensively used in matters related to addiction, especially religious abuse, this book is an important intertwining of addiction, recovery, and spiritual well-being.*

Keller, John. *Ministering to Alcoholics.* Minneapolis, MN: Augsburg Fortress, 1991.

> *A timeless authority on matters related to addiction, with particular attention to the unique opportunities presented to clergy and other ministers of health care.*

Index

T - #0497 - 101024 - C0 - 212/152/16 - PB - 9780789016188 - Gloss Lamination